NUTRITIONAL ASSESSMENT IN CRITICAL CARE
A Training Handbook

By

Donald C. Zavala, M.D., F.A.C.P., F.C.C.P.
Professor of Medicine
Department of Internal Medicine
Pulmonary Disease Division
College of Medicine
The University of Iowa
Iowa City, Iowa 52242 U.S.A.

1989

Composed at The University of Iowa, Iowa City, Iowa 52242

Nutritional Assessment in Critical Care: A Training Handbook
©1989 by Donald C. Zavala, First Edition

Copyright under the International Copyright Union. All rights reserved. This book is protected by copyright. No part of it may be reproduced, stored in a retrieval system or transmitted in any form or by any means, electronic or mechanical, including photocopying, recording, or otherwise, without written permission from the copyright owner. Made in the United States of America. Iowa City, Iowa 52242 U.S.A.

Library of Congress Cataloging-in-Publication Data
Zavala, Donald C. (Donald Charles), 1923–
    Nutritional assessment in critical care: a training handbook/ by Donald C. Zavala.—1st ed.
    Includes bibliographical references.
    ISBN 0-87414-071-4
    1. Nutrition—Evaluation. 2. Critical care medicine.
[1. Critical Care—handbooks. 2. Diet Therapy—handbooks.
3. Nutritional Requirements—handbooks. 4. Parenteral Feeding—handbooks.] I. Title.
    [DNLM: WB   39   Z39n]
RC621.Z38   1989
615.8′54—dc20
DNLM/DLC   89–5236
for Library of Congress   CIP

Note: The illustration on the front cover is an artist's drawing which demonstrates insertion of a silastic catheter for prolonged TPN (p. 87). Indirect calorimetry is utilized for determining REE and RQ.

CONTENTS

	Page
FOREWORD	ix
PREFACE	xi
ACKNOWLEDGMENTS	xiii

CHAPTER 1
Nutritional Assessment: Background Information — 1

CHAPTER 2
Evaluating Nutritional Needs:
Anthropometry, Laboratory Tests — 12

CHAPTER 3
Evalutating Nutritional Needs:
Prediction Equations, Indirect Calorimetry — 35

CHAPTER 4
Feeding the Patient: Nutritional Therapy — 67

CHAPTER 5
Comments of Clinical Importance — 112

SUMMARY — 127

REFERENCES — 130

INDEX — 144

OUTLINE

FOREWORD

PREFACE

ACKNOWLEDGMENTS

CHAPTER 1
  NUTRITIONAL ASSESSMENT
   Background Information
    -Introduction
    -Definition of Terms
    -Four Major Considerations

CHAPTER 2
  EVALUATING NUTRITIONAL NEEDS
  Part I: Anthropometry
   Fat and Muscle Status
    -Percent of Ideal Body Weight (% IBW)
    -Percent of Usual Body Weight
    -Body Mass Index
    -Triceps Skinfold (TSF)
    -Midarm Circumference (MAC)
    -Midarm Muscle Circumference (MAMC)
    -Creatinine-Height Index (CHI)

  Part II: Laboratory Tests
   Visceral Protein Status
    -Serum Albumin
    -Total Iron Binding Capacity (TIBC)
    -Transferrin
    -Other Plasma Proteins
    -Total Lymphocyte Count
    -Skin Testing for Anergy

Nitrogen Balance
　　Serum Phosphorus
　　Serum Magnesium
　　Miscellaneous

CHAPTER 3
　EVALUATING NUTRITIONAL NEEDS
　Part III: Prediction Equations for Energy Requirements
　　Equations, Calculations, Formulas
　　　-Long's Calculations
　　　-Quebbeman-Ausman Regression Equation
　　　-Regression Equation Based on Body Surface Area
　　　-Krause-Mahan Calculations for TEE
　　　-Harris-Benedict Equation
　　　-Moore-Angelillo Equation
　　　-Curreri Formula
　　　-Other Prediction Guidelines

　Part IV: Indirect Calorimetry
　　Introduction
　　Calculations
　　　-Weir's Equation
　　　-Weir's Abbreviated Equation
　　Calorimetry at the Bedside
　　　-Measurement Conditions
　　　-Operation and Quality Control
　　　-Equipment
　　　-Accessory Devices
　　　-Mechanically Ventilated Patients
　　　-Sources of Error
　　Case Study

CHAPTER 4
　FEEDING THE PATIENT: NUTRITIONAL THERAPY
　Introduction
　Enteral Nutrition
　　Nasoenteric Tube Feeding
　　　-Indications
　　　-Contraindications
　　　-Techniques
　　　-Complications
　　　-Preventive Measures

    Gastrostomy (PEG/PEJ)
    Monitoring the Patient/Tidbits
    Enteral Formulas
     -Polymeric
     -Oligomeric
     -Modular
     -Special
       Hepatic/Renal Failure
       Stress, Trauma, Burns
       Respiratory Failure
       Diabetes/Pancreatitis
       Cardiac Cachexia
     -Complete vs Incomplete

Parenteral Nutrition
    Historical Background
    Intravenous Nutrition
     -Peripheral Venous (PVN)
     -Central Venous (TPN)
       Indications
       Techniques
       Cannulation
       Catheter Care/Complications
       Extended TPN
       Complications

Management of Fluid, Electrolyte, & Acid-Base Problems
    Fluid Balance
    Chemical Balance
    Sodium/Chloride
    Hypernatremia
    Hyponatremia
    Potassium
    Calcium
    Acid-Base Balance

Parenteral Formulas/Infusions
    Energy Sources
    Formula Concentrations
    Nutrient Requirements, Infusion Rates
     -Carbohydrate (CHO)
     -Protein (PRO)
     -FAT
    Additives (to TPN Solutions)
     -Electrolytes

    -Vitamins
    -Heparin/Insulin
    -Minerals/Trace Metals
  Solutions, Techniques, Procedures
    -For Peripheral Venous Nutrition (PVN)
    -For Total Parenteral Nutrition (TPN)
    -For Cycled TPN at Home
    -For Administering TPN ("Pumps")
  Calculating Parenteral Feedings
    -Steps In Preparing Formulas
    -Practical Applications
  Suggested Reading
  Marketing Companies/Products

CHAPTER 5
COMMENTS OF CLINICAL IMPORTANCE
Nutritional Screening
Metabolic Responses to Critical Illness
  Starvation
    -Combustion of Glucose
    -Glycolysis
    -Utilization of Fatty Acids and Ketones
    -Other Major Metabolic Changes
  Hypometabolism, Hypermetabolism ("Ebb and Flow" Phases)
    -Shock
    -Trauma, Sepsis, Burns
Types of Malnutrition
  Adult Marasmus (Cachexia)
  Adult Kwashiorkor (Protein Starvation)
  Marasmus-Kwashiorkor Mixture
Potpourri
  Anthropometry
  Energy, Fuel, Starvation
  Protein (PRO), Nitrogen Balance
  Lipid Emulsions (FAT)
  Vitamins, Minerals, Water, Osmolarity
  Respiratory Quotient (RQ)
  Drug Reactions and Interactions
  Nutritional Assessment
Team Approach

SUMMARY

FOREWORD

The physiologic stress of illness places a great demand on a person's requirements for nutrients. The issue of how much nutritional support to provide, based on individual differences and the disease state, has been cause of debate. Historically, calorie provisions were based on formula calculations. New advances in technology have made bedside measurements of actual energy expenditure practical and reliable. Dr. Zavala, through his extensive knowledge of the physiology of gas exchange and its relationship to nutrition, provides a clear explanation of nutritional assessment in critically ill patients. By precisely measuring a patient's energy requirements, the practitioner can avoid over infusing unnecessary calories as well as inadequate nutrient delivery resulting in, or exacerbating, malnutrition. Dr. Zavala's book includes anthropometric measurements, laboratory tests, indirect calorimetry methodology, data interpretation, and nutritional prescription guidelines. His addition of a detailed case study transforms theory into practice. He has succeeded in incorporating useful information that has not been previously compiled in any other reference. This work is suitable for a variety of audiences, including those with experience in medicine seeking further knowledge of nutritional support and those with little background desiring a publication that provides the essential components of nutritional care in a hospital setting.

                          Rose Ann Sippy, MS, RD
                          Director, Dietary Department
                          University of Iowa Hospitals and Clinics
                          Iowa City, Iowa 52242

PREFACE

Almost two years ago, I began this effort as an outgrowth of my involvement in exercise physiology, with the ultimate goal of integrating the basic concepts of nutritional assessment into our training program at The University of Iowa College of Medicine.

When computerized metabolic carts (mobile units equipped with oxygen and carbon dioxide gas analyzers) first appeared on the scene, I was struck by the similarity of this equipment to the set-up in our stress testing laboratory. In fact, with only minor modifications (chiefly in software), our instruments could be used to carry out resting metabolic measurements. Furthermore, I was captivated by the concept of converting O_2 uptake ($\dot{V}O_2$) and CO_2 production ($\dot{V}CO_2$) into resting energy expenditure (kilocalories/day) and, in addition, utilizing the respiratory quotient ($\dot{V}CO_2/\dot{V}O_2$) to determine the proper mixture of substrate for fuel—an improvement over the method of estimating kilocalories by the Harris-Benedict equation. Subsequently, mobile metabolic monitors have proven to be useful in critical care situations (e.g., extensive burns, multiple trauma, sepsis) where overfeeding, underfeeding, and incorrect fuel mixtures can be major problems.

Thus, the desire to write a basic, training handbook was born! But by no stretch of the imagination is this an extensive work nor is it meant to be. After organizing my thoughts into writing, I soon realized that I had a tiger by the tail. Therefore, it should be no surprise that this book never would have been possible without the help, careful review, and suggestions of my colleagues who are actively involved in the nutritional care of sick patients (see Acknowledgments). The end result was a systematic approach to the subject, starting with a definition of terms, then proceeding to anthropometry, laboratory tests, prediction equations, indirect calorimetry at the bedside, and finally ending with information on feeding malnourished and stressed patients. I certainly hope that this pragmatic approach will be helpful to students, technicians, dietitians, nurses, and physicians in training or private practice.

I recognize that nutrition is a rapidly changing field and that some of the information in this book may be outdated in a short time. I welcome the comments of readers that may prove to be useful in future modifications and revisions of this text. Upon finishing this introductory teaching handbook, it is hoped that the reader will proceed to explore the literature further. For additional reading, I strongly recommend starting with the following two authoritative, first-class books that I am sure will serve as excellent references for some time to come:

(1) Bernard MA, Jacobs DO, Rombeau JL (eds): *Nutritional and Metabolic Support of Hospitalized Patients,* Philadelphia, WB Saunders Co, 1986.

(2) Blackburn GL, Bell SJ, Mullen JL (eds): *Nutritional Medicine, A Case Management Approach,* Philadelphia, WB Saunders Co, 1989.

And finally, good luck to all of you who wish to improve your skills in nutritional assessment!

Donald C. Zavala, M.D.
Iowa City, Iowa, U.S.A.

ACKNOWLEDGMENTS

This handbook would not have been possible without the fine diagnostic facilities provided at The University of Iowa Hospitals and Clinics or without the ideal academic environment created by Dr. Francois M. Abboud, Professor and Head of the Department of Medicine, and Dr. Gary Hunninghake, Professor and Director of the Pulmonary Division.

The author is deeply indebted to the following individuals with specialized knowledge who took their valuable time to review this handbook with care and to offer many helpful suggestions. Such colleagues play a vital, behind-the-scenes role in the making of an educational book.

(1) Adel S. Al-Jurf, M.B., Ch.B.
    Professor of Surgery
    The University of Iowa College of Medicine

(2) Lloyd J. Filer, M.D., Ph.D.
    Professor Emeritus
    Department of Pediatrics
    The University of Iowa College of Medicine

(3) Douglas Morgan, R.Ph., M.S.
    Clinical Pharmacy Specialist
    Department of Pharmacy
    The University of Iowa Hospitals and Clinics

(4) Lewis D. Stegink, Ph.D.
    Professor of Biochemistry and Pediatrics
    The University of Iowa College of Medicine

(5) Ellen F. Wade, R.D., L.D.
    Critical Care Dietitian
    Dietary Department
    The University of Iowa Hospitals and Clinics

(6) Joel V. Weinstock, M.D.
    Associate Professor of Medicine
    Director, Division of Gastroenterology-Hepatology
    The University of Iowa College of Medicine

                                                    DCZ

BOOK ORDER INFORMATION

All proceeds from this edition are being placed in a special account, Department of Medicine, The University of Iowa College of Medicine.

ORDERS (check, money order, or institutional purchase order) should be made out to:
Department of Medicine, U. of Iowa

AND SENT TO:
Louis Eichler
Publication Order Service
M 105 Oakdale Hall
The University of Iowa
Iowa City, Iowa 52242 U.S.A.

CHAPTER 1
NUTRITIONAL ASSESSMENT
Background Information

Introduction

As illustrated in Figure 1, page 2, the amount of energy used by a healthy person during rest (asleep and awake) accounts for approximately 70% of the total energy expended by the individual over 24 hours, with the balance consisting of physical activity and a rise in heat produced by the body after eating.[1] Specifically, dietary thermogenesis of normal oral diets is about 10% above the postabsorptive resting energy expenditure (REE) over 24 hours,[2] with the effect peaking within the first hour after a light meal and returning to baseline within the next hour.[3] Under normal conditions, the basal metabolic rate (BMR) represents 90% of the REE,[2] and energy expenditure during sleep decreases to around 80% of the resting level.[4] After basal needs, physical activity is the greatest single factor influencing the energy needs of a healthy person and may vary from as little as 10% of the total energy requirement (bedridden person) to as high as 50% in an athlete.[5]

Food provides the fuel for the human body to meet these energy requirements (Table 1), with the combustion of one gram of carbohydrate (CHO) yielding 4.0 calories, one gram of protein (PRO) 4.0 Calories and one gram of fat (FAT) 9.0 Calories.* Whereas CHO and FAT are converted entirely to CO_2 and H_2O in the presence of oxygen, PRO is not completely oxidized and yields CO_2, H_2O, and urea. The respiratory quotients (RQs) produced from CHO, PRO, and FAT are 1.0, 0.82, and 0.71 respectively (Table 1). Thus, to maintain a normal metabolic state in a healthy person, the intake of food

---

*These values are commonly used in calculating the energy (kcals) in ingested food, although the figures are not absolutely exact. For example, one gram of fat is closer to 9.1 Calories.

EXPENDITURE OF ENERGY IN HEALTHY INDIVIDUALS OVER 24 HOURS

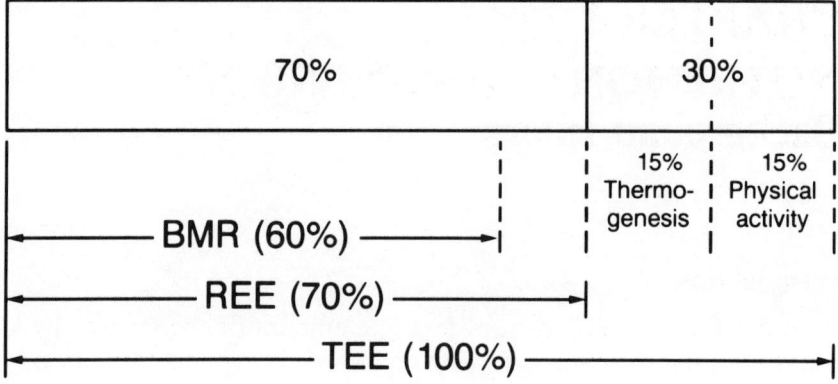

Figure 1. The approximate amount of energy expended in a normal person is shown under different conditions (basal, resting, thermogenesis, physical activity) as a percentage of the total energy expended during 24 hours. The energy needs for physical activity may vary widely from person to person. BMR = basal metabolic rate, REE = resting energy expenditure, and TEE = total energy expenditure.

(exogenous calories) must be balanced against the total amount of energy expended, otherwise body weight will change.[6] The energy balance relationship is illustrated in Figure 2, page 4.

In illness or injury, the additional nutritional needs of patients may vary widely and must be evaluated on an individual basis. For example, persons with mild to moderate chronic obstructive lung disease (COPD) may be only mildly hypermetabolic with adequate energy stores and muscle mass while other patients with severe trauma, sepsis, burns, or malignancies may be extremely hypermetabolic, catabolic, and severely nutritionally depleted. Therefore, the objectives of an exemplary nutritional program are to meet the level of stress, prevent protein loss (lean body mass), and avoid under- or overfeeding. Not only must body tissue and energy reserves be restored (anabolism), but also the resting energy expenditure (REE), coupled with increased energy demands brought on by injury or disease, must be met and maintained[7] (Figure 3). To further compound the problem, patients in critical care situations often are unable to take food via the gastrointestinal tract and must be fed parenterally.

Table 1. FUEL VALUE AND RQ OF MAJOR NUTRIENTS

Substrate	Heat of Combustion in Bomb Calorimeter (Cal/g)	Physiologic Fuel Value (Cal/g)	Respiratory Quotient (RQ)
Ethanol	7.1	7.0	0.67
Fats	9.45	9.0	0.71
Protein	5.65	4.0	0.82
Carbohydrates	4.1	4.0	1.0
Balanced diet	6.21	5.75	0.87
OTHER SITUATIONS			
Overfeeding (lipogenesis)	–	–	1.0–1.2
Starvation	–	–	0.65–0.67
Hypoventilation	–	–	0.71
Hyperventilation	–	–	>1.0

NOTE: Substrate data (except for balanced diet) was taken from Anderson CE: Energy and metabolism. *In* Schneider HA, Anderson CE, Coursin DB (eds), *Nutritional Support of Medical Practice*. Haggerstown, MD, Harper & Row Publishers, 1977, p. 11, with permission. The balanced diet consists of 50% CHO, 15% PRO, and 35% FAT.

To achieve the goal of adequate nutrition under trying conditions, it is essential that the patient's nutritional status be carefully appraised and that the total energy needs and proper substrate mix (CHO, PRO, FAT) be accurately determined. The best approach is the use of anthropometry, selected laboratory tests, and indirect calorimetry. By no means does the author intend to present an extensive, detailed discussion but rather to summarize the topic and to furnish the reader with pertinent references for a more thorough review.

Definition of Terms

It is important for the reader to have an understanding of the following terms commonly used in discussions relating to nutritional assessment. The terms are grouped according to the subject matter.

Body Metabolism: **the process of converting foodstuffs into energy.** The chemical energy of ingested food cannot be used directly but requires ATP (adenosine triphosphate), which acts as an "energetic inter-

Nutritional Assessment

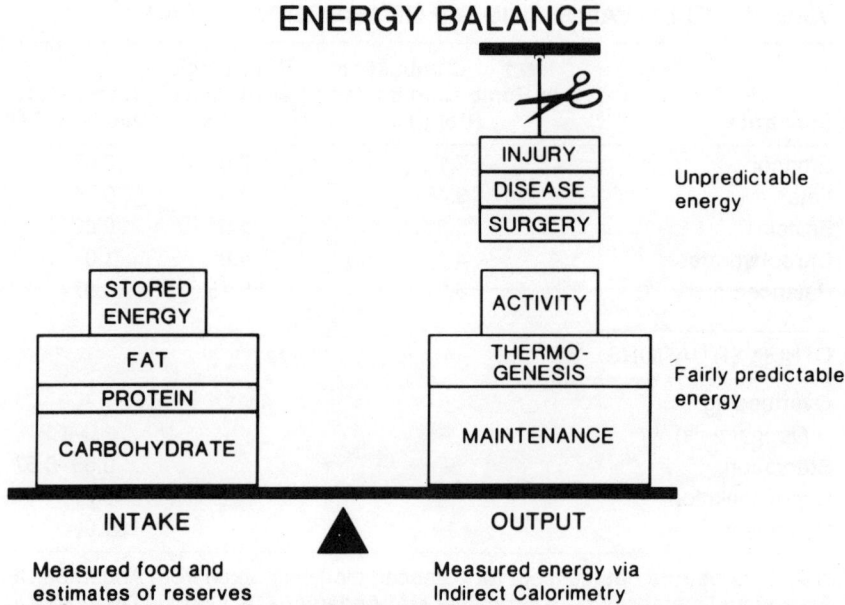

Figure 2. The balance of energy (intake vs output) is illustrated in health and disease. Adapted from French SN[1] with permission.

mediary." Oxidation of the ingested substrate occurs at the cellular level (cellular respiration) by decarboxylation and by the gradual removal of hydrogen and pairs of electrons of food molecules via the mitochondrial respiratory chain. At the end of the cycle, the hydrogen and electrons are united with molecules of O_2 to form H_2O. During this process the bond energies of food molecules are released and captured in forming high-energy ATP from adenosine diphosphate (ADP) that is present in cell fluid. The combined process of the respiratory cycle and the transfer of electrons from food to molecular oxygen with the forming of ATP is termed coupled oxidative phosphorylation. The reader is referred to Lehninger's definition of cellular respiration in *Biochemistry,* New York, Worth Publishers, Inc., 1970, p. 337.

Nutritional Assessment

RESTING ENERGY EXPENDITURE

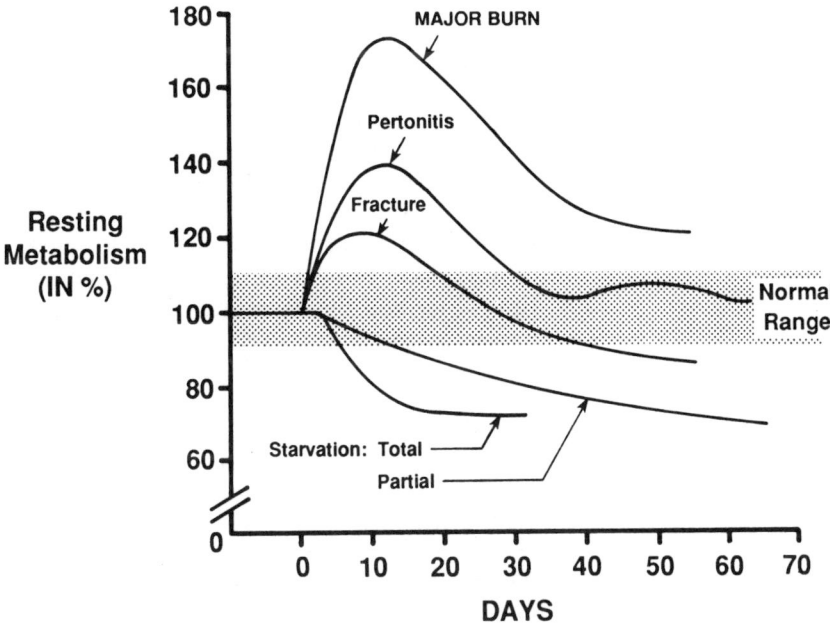

Figure 3. Changes in REE (expressed in percent of normal range) is shown, demonstrating increases in hypermetabolic or **flow** states (burns, trauma, infection) and decreases in hypometabolic or **ebb** states (starvation, also shock). From Long CL, et al[7], with permission.

Anabolism: the process of building up tissues and energy reserve (constructive metabolism).

Catabolism: the process of breaking down tissues and energy reserve (destructive metabolism).

Gluconeogenesis: the formation of new glucose from noncarbohydrate precursors, lactate being one of the most important.[8]

Substrate: the type of substance or food (carbohydrate [CHO], protein [PRO], or fat [FAT]) from which energy is available. For the activities of daily living, this energy is stored and transferred in the form of high-energy phosphate bonds.

Nutritional Assessment

Thermogenesis: **the production of heat by a living organism.** There are three types of thermogenesis.

(1) **Essential** thermogenesis refers to the heat generated by the maintenance of cellular functions in the body, including anabolic and catabolic reactions.

(2) **Dietary** thermogenesis refers to the increase in heat production resulting from a rise in the rate of body metabolism following the intake of nutrients. This thermic effect of food was first described by Rubner as a "specific dynamic action" that varies according to the amount and type of substrate ingested.[9]

(3) **Shivering** thermogenesis involves skeletal muscle, resulting in an increase in heat production (and heat loss) caused by exposure to cold temperatures.[2]

Anthropometry: **the science that deals with comparative measurements of the human body,** for example, height, weight, triceps skinfold, upper midarm circumference, wrist circumference, and so forth. Ideally, *height* is taken with the subject standing in stocking feet against a straight surface (e.g., stadiometer). One also may use a vertical measuring rod with the head held erect. Routinely, *weight* is obtained on a standard, balanced beam scale with the subject dressed in underwear or a gown. The aim of anthropemetry in critical care is to identify undernourished, and severely malnourished patients as easily as possible. Follow up measurements during the course of illness are of value.

Body Surface Area: the area of the exterior surface of the body that
(BSA) can be calculated using a formula developed by DuBois:[10] Surface area (m²) = .007184 × $W^{0.425}$ × $H^{0.725}$, where m² = square meters, W = weight in kg, and H = height in cm. This formula has an average error of only 1.7% for adults but is not valid for children under 6 years of age.

Lean Body Mass: (LBM)	the portion of the body that is nonfat and is composed of skeleton, muscle, viscera, plasma proteins, extracellular fluid, and skin.[11]
Calorimetry:	**Direct calorimetry is the measurement of whole-body heat loss** that is carried out in a specially designed, insulated chamber with coils in its walls. The temperature in the chamber is kept constant while heat produced by the subject is absorbed by water circulating in the coils. Measurements include the increase in water temperature, flow rate of the water, and water vapor in the exhaled breath. Although accurate, the procedure is complicated and unwieldy. **Indirect calorimetry involves the measurement of gas exchange** whereby oxygen uptake ($\dot{V}O_2$) and carbon dioxide production ($\dot{V}CO_2$) are readily utilized to determine the amount of energy expended in the body and the respiratory quotient (RQ). The energy production (caloric value) of O_2 is a function of the type of substrate or mixtures being oxidized (RQ) and is expressed as kcal/unit time (see Weir's equation, p. 42). For each kcal of CHO metabolized, 200 ml of O_2 is consumed and 200 ml of CO_2 is produced (RQ = 200/200 = 1.0). For each kcal of PRO metabolized, RQ = 190 ml CO_2/240 ml O_2 = 0.8. For one kcal of FAT metabolized, RQ = 150 ml CO_2/200 ml O_2 = 0.7.
$\dot{V}O_2$:	**oxygen uptake** (ml/min or ml/kg/min).
$\dot{V}CO_2$:	**carbon dioxide output** (ml/min).
RQ:	**the respiratory quotient** = $\dot{V}CO_2/\dot{V}O_2$, in the steady state. At rest, this gas exchange ratio reflects the substrate mixture (fuel) being metabolized (see Table 1, p. 3).
RQ_{NP}:	**the non-protein respiratory quotient:** $$RQ_{NP} = \frac{\dot{V}CO_2 \text{ ml/min} - 4.8 \text{ UN}}{\dot{V}O_2 \text{ ml/min} - 5.9 \text{ UN}}, \text{ where}$$ UN = total urinary nitrogen in grams/day.

Nutritional Assessment

MET: the metabolic equivalent of an individual, which is a convenient way of defining levels of physical activity:

$$MET = \frac{\dot{V}O_2 \text{ (measured)}}{\dot{V}O_2 \text{ (at rest)}}$$

The average oxygen uptake at rest = 3.5 ml/kg/min or 1.0 MET; driving a car = 1.5 METs (5.25 ml O_2/kg/min); and walking 3 miles/hour = 3 METs (10.5 ml O_2/kg/min).

Kilocalorie: (kcal or Cal) the amount of heat needed to raise the temperature of one kilogram of water by one degree Celsius, from 15° C to 16° C. A kilocalorie (Calorie with a capital **C**) is equal to 1000 small calories spelled with a lower case **c**. To convert kilocalories (a measure of thermal energy) to kilojoules (a measure of mechanical energy), multiply the number of kilocalories by 4.2 (4.184, to be exact).[12]

Calorie/Nitrogen: (Cal/N) a ratio that is used to ascertain whether Calories and protein (PRO) are being delivered at suitable levels.[7,13]

The ratio is calculated as follows: $\frac{\text{Cal/day}}{\text{N (g/day)}}$, where $N = \frac{\text{PRO (g)}}{6.25}$.

For moderately to severely stressed patients, the recommended ratio is 150:1 with a range of 180:1 to 120:1. For normal body maintenance, ratios of 250 to 300 kcal/g N are appropriate. **Note:** Values for *nonprotein calories (NPC/g N)* sometimes are used instead of total Calories, with a range of 100:1 to 80:1 for moderately to severely stressed patients. For normal body maintenance the ratio is 150:1.

Osmolarity: the osmotic concentration of a solute (the dissolved substance in a solution), expressed as osmols of solute/L. See page 121 for a further discussion of osmolarity.

Nutritional Assessment

Energy Requirements: **the daily energy needs of the individual.** The number of Calories expended for various daily activities are listed below.[14]

DAILY ENERGY NEEDS:

ACTIVITY	MEN (Cal/kg/hr)	WOMEN (Cal/kg/hr)
Very Light: driving, typing, standing	1.5	1.3
Light: walking 2.5–3 mph, golf, carpentry, tennis	2.9	2.6
Moderate: walking 3.5–4 mph, hoeing, dancing, cycling	4.3	4.1
Heavy: pick and shovel work, climbing, swimming, football	8.4	8.0

Note: The above mean values were adapted from RDA (Recommended Daily Dietary Allowances) published by the National Research Council, Food and Nutrition Board, 9th edition, 1980. Adjustments have not been made for height, weight, or age. Other tables are readily available that list the metabolic cost of various occupational and leisure activities.[15] If the data are expressed as ml's of O_2/kg/min, then these values can be converted (an approximation) to Cal/kg/hour as follows:

$$\text{Cal/kg/hr} = \frac{7.2 \times \text{ml } O_2/\text{kg/min}}{24} \quad \text{(see p. 43)}.$$

BEE: **the basal energy expenditure of the individual.** In the original studies, this measurement was *not* carried out in a basal state upon awakening (like a BMR) but instead was done under resting conditions anytime during the day similar to REE (see below).[16] Thus, BEE is equivalent to REE values, but the term REE is preferred since it more accurately describes the conditions of the test.

Nutritional Assessment

BMR: **the basal metabolic rate of the individual.** This measurement of body metabolism represents the minimal amount of heat produced, that is, the minimal amount of energy required to sustain the organism. Traditionally, the test is performed in the early morning within 30 minutes upon awakening, 12 to 18 hours after the ingestion of food.[3] The subject is at complete muscular rest and in a comfortable environment.

REE: **the resting energy expenditure of the individual.** This measurement, which is approximately 10% higher than the BMR, is taken any time during the day at least 2 hours postprandially to avoid the acute, thermic effect of food.[3] Prior to testing, the subject should be in a resting state for at least 30 minutes and have no skeletal movement during the test.

TEE: **the total energy expenditure of the individual.** This measurement includes the sum of energy expenditure (EE) during sleep, rest, thermogenesis, and physical activity.

CVN: **central venous nutrition.** This route of nourishment indicates that concentrated nutrient solutions (dextrose, amino acids, fat emulsions, and additives) are given via the superior vena cava. The usual access route is through the subclavian or internal jugular vein.

PVN: **peripheral venous nutrition,** also called peripheral parenteral nutrition, indicates that the feedings are given by peripheral vein rather than by central vein. The solutions may provide up to 2000–2200 kcal/day. By itself, PVN is appropriate for patients who have only minor or moderate nutritional defects or needs over a short period of time.

TPN: **total parenteral nutrition.** The required nutrients (amino acids, dextrose, lipid emulsions, vitamins, minerals) are given by vein rather than via the gastrointestinal tract. Usually a central vein is utilized, but in special, short-term situations the route may be by peripheral vein. The purpose of TPN is to meet **all** of the maintenance and stress requirements of the patient. In addition to bowel rest, adequate parenteral nutrition will replenish the malnourished patient.[17]

FOUR MAJOR CONSIDERATIONS

When evaluating the nutritional needs of an injured or ill patient, there are four major considerations to take into account:

(1) Anthropometry

(2) Laboratory tests

(3) Prediction equations

(4) Indirect calorimetry

With the introduction and refinement of mobile metabolic carts, indirect calorimetry is augmenting prediction equations as an exceptionally accurate method to determine the patient's resting energy expenditure (REE). Now let us proceed to the vitally important, fascinating subject of nutritional assessment in critical care.

CHAPTER 2
EVALUATING NUTRITIONAL NEEDS

PART I: ANTHROPOMETRY (Table 2)*

Fat and Muscle Status *(see adult marasmus, p. 116).* The percent of ideal body weight (% IBW), percent of usual body weight, body mass index, and triceps skinfold (TSF) serve as indicators of body fat stores. On the other hand, the patient's muscle mass is approximated from measurements of midarm circumference (MAC), midarm muscle circumference (MAMC), and creatinine-height index (CHI).

(1) Percent of Ideal Body Weight (% IBW). The patient's current, actual weight is expressed as a percent of his or her ideal weight:

$$\% \text{ IBW} = \frac{\text{current weight}}{\text{ideal weight}} \times 100, \text{ where}$$

IBW = ideal body weight, which can be determined using the normograms shown in Tables 3 and 4, or a rule-of-thumb calculation in Table 5.

Based on the percent of ideal body weight, the degree of malnutrition may be classified as follows:[18]

80–90% = mild malnutrition
60–80% = moderate malnutrition
 <60% = severe malnutrition

---

*Note: Anthropometry consists of **indirect estimates** of fat and muscle (protein) stores. The major factors affecting the reliability of anthropometry are as follows: (1) Rapid changes in extracellular water may invalidate body weight as an index of cell mass, (2) There may be significant variability in interobserver measurements, especially among inexperienced personnel, and (3) Acute changes in the patient's status are not reflected in certain measurements (e.g., triceps skinfold, midarm circumference, and midarm muscle circumference).

Table 2. NUTRITIONAL ASSESSMENT

BODY SYSTEM	MEASUREMENT
Fat Stores	Triceps Skinfold*
	% Ideal or Usual Weight*
Protein Status	Nitrogen Balance
viscera	Serum Albumin
	Total Iron Binding Capacity
	Transferrin
	Total Lymphocyte Count
	Skin Tests for Anergy
skeletal muscle	Midarm Circumference*
	Midarm Muscle Circumference*
	Creatinine-Height Index*
Metabolic Status	Prediction Equations
(Calories needed)	Indirect Calorimetry

NOTE: Anthropometric measurements for fat stores and skeletal muscle are indicated by an asterisk (*). The laboratory studies shown above are used to evaluate the status of visceral protein. Nitrogen (N) balance measures N (in) −N (out).

(2) **Percent of Usual Body Weight.** The patient's current weight is expressed as a percent of his or her usual weight.[19]

$$\% \text{ Usual Weight} = \frac{\text{current weight}}{\text{usual weight}} \times 100.$$

Thus, based on the % of usual body weight:

85–95% = mild malnutrition
75–85% = moderate malnutrition
<75% = severe malnutrition

Note: *In the clinical setting, body weight may be significantly affected by the patient's status of hydration (e.g. dehydration vs. edema, extracellular water).* Disease states such as congestive heart failure, renal failure, or hepatic failure with ascites can greatly alter body weight. Also, fluid overload will rapidly increase the patient's weight.

(3) **Body Mass Index (BMI).** The BMI is a useful calculation to estimate the fat compartment of the body, especially when used along with skinfold measurements (see below). The values obtained may be greatly affected by the patient's degree of hydration as stated

Evaluating Nutritional Needs

Table 3.

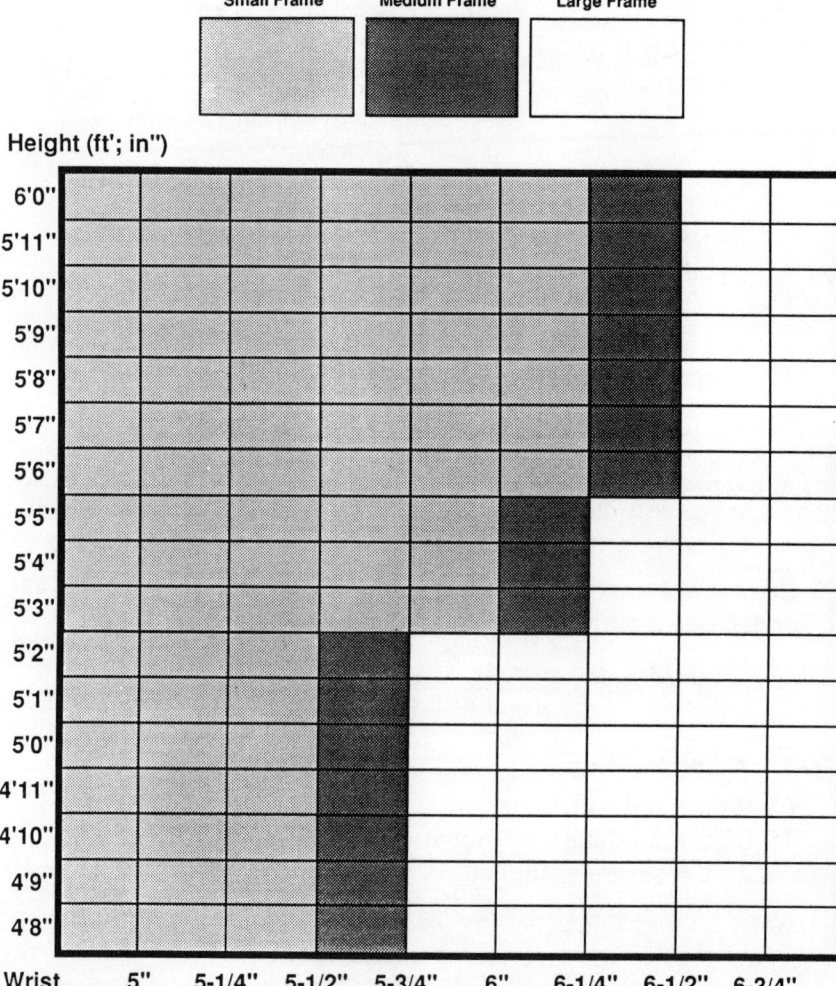

NOTE: The wrist is measured in inches, distal to the styloid process of the radius and ulna at the smallest circumference. The height is measured in inches without shoes.
Source: Anne Grant, *Nutritional Guidelines,* Seattle, Washington, 1979, p. 7. Reprinted with permission. Also see Grant A, DeHoog S: *Nutritional Assessment and Support,* 3rd edition, Box 75057, Seattle, Washington 98125, 1985, p. 7.

Table 4. IDEAL WEIGHT (kg) FOR HEIGHT: ADULTS*

	MALES			FEMALES		
cm	Small Frame	Medium Frame	Large Frame	Small Frame	Medium Frame	Large Frame
142				41.8	45.0	49.5
143				42.3	45.3	49.8
144				42.8	45.6	50.1
145				43.2	45.9	50.5
146				43.7	46.6	51.2
147				44.1	47.3	51.8
148				44.6	47.7	52.3
149				45.1	48.1	52.8
150				45.5	48.6	53.2
151				46.2	49.3	54.0
152				46.8	50.0	54.5
153				47.3	50.5	55.0
154				47.8	51.0	55.5
155	50.0	53.6	58.2	48.2	51.4	55.9
156	50.7	54.3	58.8	48.9	52.3	56.8
157	51.4	55.0	59.5	49.5	53.2	57.7
158	51.8	55.5	60.0	50.0	53.6	58.3
159	52.2	56.0	60.5	50.5	54.0	58.9
160	52.7	56.4	60.9	50.9	54.5	59.5
161	53.2	56.8	61.5	51.5	55.3	60.1
162	53.7	57.2	62.1	52.1	56.1	60.7
163	54.1	57.7	62.7	52.7	56.8	61.4
164	55.0	58.5	63.4	53.6	57.7	62.3
165	55.9	59.5	64.1	54.5	58.6	63.2
166	56.5	60.1	64.8	55.1	59.2	63.8
167	57.1	60.7	65.6	55.7	59.8	64.4
168	57.7	61.4	66.4	56.4	60.5	65.0
169	58.6	62.3	67.5	57.3	61.4	65.9
170	59.5	63.2	68.6	58.2	62.2	66.8
171	60.1	63.8	69.2	58.8	62.8	67.4
172	60.7	64.4	69.8	59.4	63.4	68.0
173	61.4	65.0	70.5	60.0	64.1	68.6
174	62.3	65.9	71.4	60.9	65.0	69.8
175	63.2	66.8	72.3	61.8	65.9	70.9
176	63.8	67.5	72.9	62.4	66.5	71.7
177	64.4	68.2	73.5	63.0	67.1	72.5
178	65.0	69.0	74.1	63.6	67.7	73.2

continued

Evaluating Nutritional Needs

Table 4.   IDEAL WEIGHT (kg) FOR HEIGHT: ADULTS* continued

	MALES			FEMALES		
cm	Small Frame	Medium Frame	Large Frame	Small Frame	Medium Frame	Large Frame
179	65.9	69.9	75.3	64.5	68.6	74.1
180	66.8	70.9	76.4	65.5	69.5	75.0
181	67.4	71.7	77.1	66.1	70.1	75.6
182	68.0	72.5	77.8	66.7	70.7	76.2
183	68.6	73.2	78.6	67.3	71.4	76.8
184	69.8	74.1	79.8			
185	70.9	75.0	80.9			
186	71.5	75.8	81.7			
187	72.1	76.6	82.5			
188	72.7	77.3	83.2			
189	73.3	78.0	83.8			
190	73.9	78.7	84.4			
191	74.5	79.5	85.0			

*These tables correct for the 1969 Metropolitan Life Insurance Co. standards to height without shoes and weight without clothes. Derived from data of the 1969 Build and Blood Pressure Study, Society of Actuaries.

above. The formula for BMI divides the weight of the subject in kilograms by the height in meters squared to estimate overall fat stores:[20] BMI = W/H^2, where W = weight in kg and H^2 = height in meters squared. By rule of thumb, the normal range is 22–27. In general, patients with a BMI less than 21 are underweight and less than 15 are severely weight depleted. On the other side of the scale,

Table 5.   RULE OF THUMB DETERMINATION FOR IDEAL BODY WEIGHT

Females:	100 lb. (45 kg.) for the first 5 ft. (152 cm), *plus* 5 lb. (2.2 kg) for every inch (2.54 cm) of height over 5 ft. (152 cm).
Males:	104 lb. (47 kg) for the first 5 ft. (152 cm), *plus* 5 lb. (2.2 kg) for every inch (2.54 cm) of height over 5 ft. (152 cm).
Example:	female, 165 cm. height, medium frame: 45 kg + (2.2 kg × 13/2.54) = 56.3 kg (ideal body weight)
Note:	To adjust for frame size, add 10 lb (4.5 kg) for a large frame or subtract 10 lb. (4.5 kg) for a small frame.

From Krause MV, Mahan LK: Food, Nutrition and Diet Therapy, 7th ed., Philadelphia, WB Saunders Co, 1984, p. 20, with permission.

an individual can be classified as obese when the body mass index is greater than 27.8 for men or 27.3 for women.[21] Increased mortality has been noted in patients with a BMI of 30 or higher, and morbid obesity is identified with values of 45 or more.

(4) Triceps Skinfold TSF.* Normally, about 50% of body fat is subcutaneous. By measuring the triceps skinfold, an indirect estimate of total body fat reserves (energy stores) can be obtained by using anthropometric data (Table 6).[22-24] The fatfold thickness is measured in millimeters at the back of the midpoint of the upper arm with a reliable caliper such as a *Lang* Skinfold Caliper (Cambridge Scientific Industries, Inc., Cambridge, MD 21613) or a *Harpenden* Skinfold Caliper (British Industries, LTD., St. Albans, Hertfordshire, England). Also, one can use a *Ross* Adipometer Skinfold Caliper (Ross Laboratories, Columbus, OH).

While standing or sitting, the subject's nondominant arm, with the elbow bent at 90° angle, should be hanging relaxed at the side. If the patient is supine, the skinfold thickness can still be measured with the arm folded across the chest. Using the thumb and index finger, the examiner gently pulls away a lengthwise skinfold from the underlying triceps muscle and places the jaws of the caliper over the skin fold (at a depth equal to the thickness of the fold) at the *midpoint mark* between the acromion (shoulder) and the olecranon (elbow). If the Adipometer Skinfold Caliper™ is used, force is exerted with the thumb and forefinger of the examiner's dominant hand until the lines of the caliper are aligned (Figure 4). If a Lang or Harpenden Caliper is employed, then pressure is necessary to open the jaws prior to placing the instrument on the skinfold. An average of three readings is taken and recorded to the nearest 1.0 mm. Percentile distributions for the triceps skinfold measurements are shown on the next page in Table 6, including standards for determining nutritional status.

(5) Midarm Circumference (MAC) and Midarm Muscle Circumference (MAMC). These two measurements serve as an index of muscle mass (somatic protein stores) and are characteristically decreased in protein malnutrition. The *midarm circumference (MAC)* is carefully measured using a nonstretchable tape, usually made of metal or fiberglass. The patient's arm should be hanging

---

*Subscapular skinfold thickness also may be used to assess body fat except on bedfast patients who cannot be turned to the side for measurement, patients who have thermal injury to the upper back, or patients who are in a body cast. Note: Lang and Harpenden calipers are the most accurate (contact pressure of $10g/mm^2$).

Evaluating Nutritional Needs

Table 6. TRICEPS SKINFOLD (mm), Males

Age (years)	Percentile						
	90th	75th	50th	25th	15th	10th	5th
18–24	20.0	14.0	9.5	7.0	6.0	5.0	4.0
25–34	21.5	16.0	12.0	8.0	6.0	5.5	4.5
35–44	20.0	15.5	12.0	8.5	7.0	6.0	5.0
45–54	20.0	15.0	11.0	8.0	7.0	6.0	5.0
55–64	18.0	14.0	11.0	8.0	6.5	6.0	5.0
65–74	19.0	15.0	11.0	8.0	6.5	5.5	4.5

TRICEPS SKINFOLD (mm), Females

Age (years)	Percentile						
	90th	75th	50th	25th	15th	10th	5th
18–24	30.0	24.0	18.0	14.0	12.0	11.0	9.4
25–34	33.5	26.5	21.0	16.0	13.5	12.0	10.5
35–44	35.5	29.5	23.0	18.0	16.0	14.0	12.0
45–54	36.5	30.0	25.0	20.0	17.0	15.0	13.0
55–64	35.0	30.5	25.0	19.0	16.0	14.0	11.0
65–74	33.0	28.0	23.0	18.0	16.0	14.0	11.5

NOTE: The above data were collected by the National Center for Health Statistics during the Health and Nutritional Examination Survey (HANES) of 1971 to 1974.[22] Age- and sex-specific percentile distributions were developed from the data by Bishop and colleagues.[23,24] Adapted from *Am J Clin Nutr* 34: 2530–2539, 1981, with permission. *The following standards apply for determining nutritional status:*[25]

    <5th percentile = Depleted
    5–15th percentile = Marginally depleted
    15–85th percentile = Normal
    >85th percentile = Above normal

loosely at the side while the examiner takes an average of three readings (in centimeters) at the midpoint of the upper arm (Figure 5). Once having accurately measured the MAC and the TSF (see item 3), these two values are utilized to calculate the *midarm muscle circumference (MAMC)*. The following equation for MAMC[23-26] assumes that the upper arm is a cylinder when actually it has an oval or elliptical shape:

MAMC = MAC − (π × TSF), where
MAMC = midarm muscle circumference in cm,
MAC   = midarm circumference in cm,
TSF   = triceps skinfold in cm, and
π = 3.14

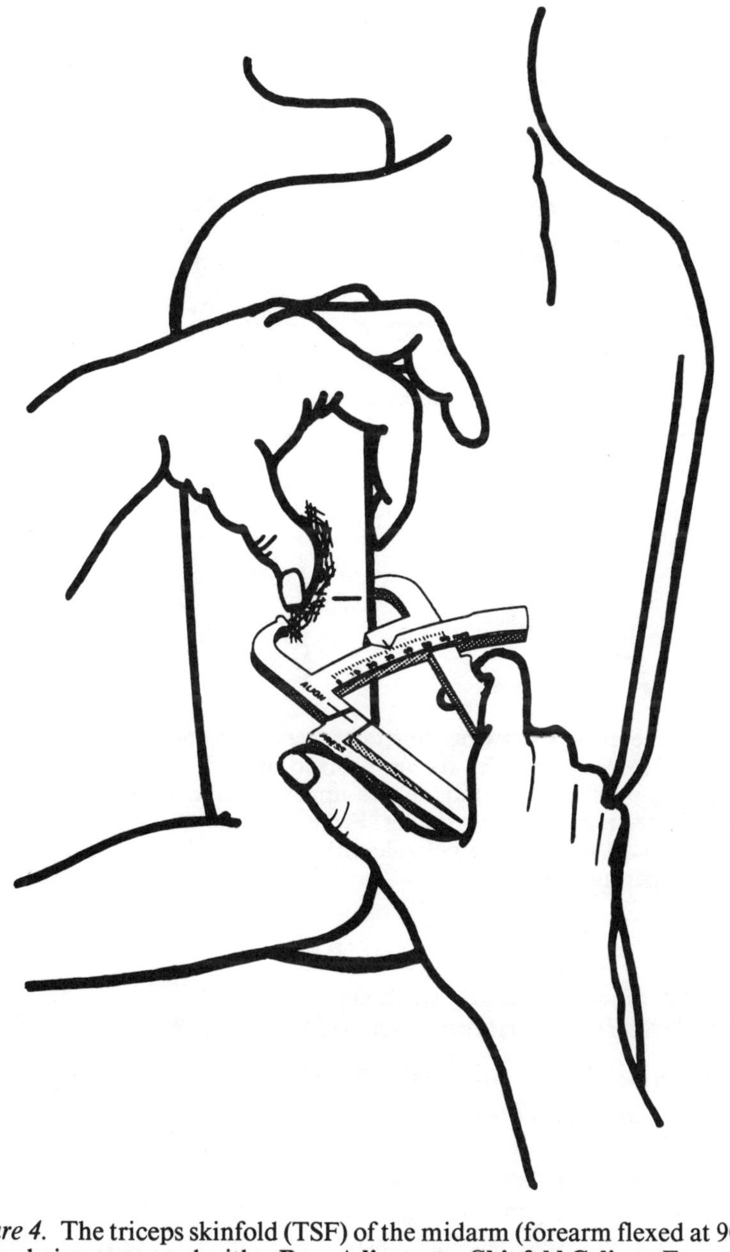

Evaluating Nutritional Needs

Figure 4. The triceps skinfold (TSF) of the midarm (forearm flexed at 90°) is shown being measured with a **Ross Adipometer Skinfold Caliper.** Force is exerted on the Adipometer until the lines of the caliper are aligned. The artist's drawing has been modified from Simko MD, Cowell C, Gilbride JA: *Nutritional Assessment,* Rockville, MD, Aspen Publishers, Inc., © 1984, p. 90, with permission.

Evaluating Nutritional Needs

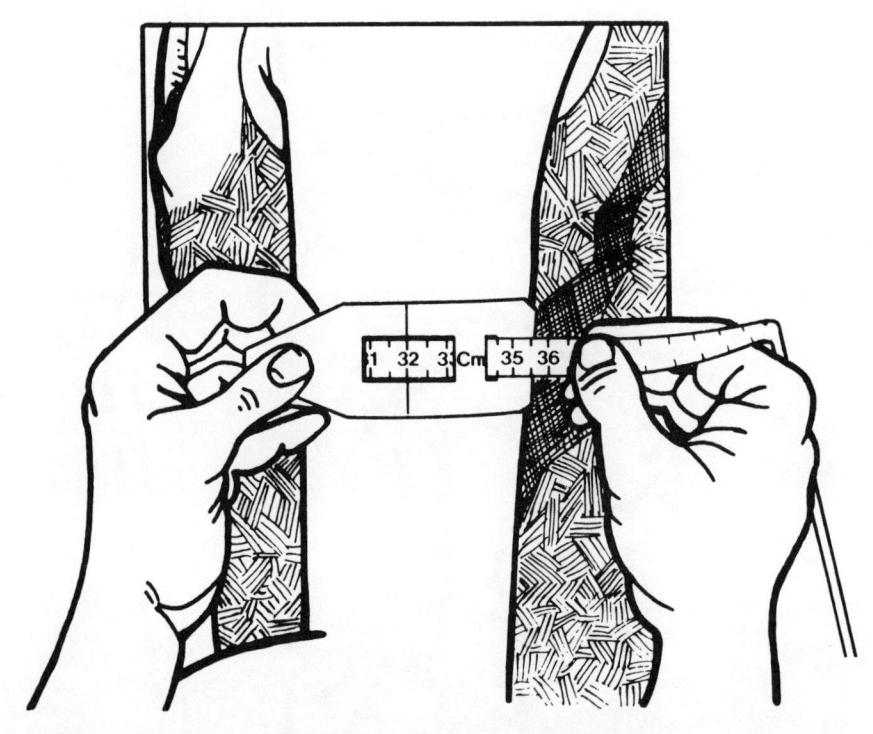

Figure 5. The artist's drawing illustrates measurement of the midarm circumference (MAC) with the forearm flexed at 90°. The **insertion tape** is drawn gently but firmly around the mid-upper arm and pulled just enough to avoid compression of the soft tissues. From Simko MD, Cowell C, Gilbride JA: *Nutritional Assessment,* Rockville, MD, Aspen Publishers, Inc., © 1984, p. 86, with permission.

Age and sex specific percentile distributions for both MAC and MAMC measurements are given in Tables 7 and 8, including standards for determining nutritional status.[22-24]

(6) Creatinine-Height Index (CHI).[*] This index involves *anthropometric and biochemical measurements,* and is an indicator of somatic protein depletion in malnourished patients.[11,18,27,28]

Both *creatinine* and *3-methylhistidine* are muscle breakdown metabolites. The measurement of 3-methylhistidine excretion is still in the research stage; however, measurement of urinary creatinine is a frequently used clinical tool. Creatine, the only pre-

[*]CHI is listed in the section on "Anthropometry" rather than "Laboratory Tests", since the values (like MAC and MAMC) reflect skeletal muscle mass.

Table 7. MIDARM CIRCUMFERENCE (cm), Males*

Age (years)	Percentile						
	90th	75th	50th	25th	15th	10th	5th
18–24	35.5	32.9	30.7	28.7	27.6	27.1	25.7
25–34	36.5	34.4	32.0	30.0	28.9	28.2	27.0
35–44	36.3	34.8	32.7	30.7	29.5	28.7	27.8
45–54	36.2	34.2	32.0	30.0	28.9	27.8	26.7
55–64	35.2	33.4	31.7	29.6	28.2	27.3	25.6
65–74	34.4	32.4	30.7	28.5	27.3	26.5	25.3

MIDARM CIRCUMFERENCE (cm), Females*

Age (years)	Percentile						
	90th	75th	50th	25th	15th	10th	5th
18–24	31.7	28.8	26.4	24.5	23.5	23.0	22.1
25–34	34.1	30.4	27.8	25.7	24.8	24.2	23.3
35–44	36.2	32.2	29.2	26.8	25.8	25.2	24.1
45–54	36.8	32.9	30.3	27.5	26.6	25.7	24.3
55–64	36.3	33.3	30.2	27.7	26.1	25.1	23.9
65–74	35.3	32.5	29.9	27.4	26.2	25.2	23.8

*Reported by Bishop, et al[23,24] from data collected during the Health and Nutritional Examination Survey (HANES) of 1971–1974.[22] Adapted from *Am J Clin Nutr* 34: 2530–2539, 1981, with permission.
The following standards apply for determining nutritional status:[25]
 <5th percentile = Depleted
 5–15th percentile = Marginally depleted
 15–85th percentile = Normal
 >85th percentile = Above normal

cursor of creatinine, is found primarily in muscle where it is irreversibly converted from creatine phosphate to creatinine and excreted in the urine in proportion to the amount of skeletal muscle in the person's body. The excretion of 1 mg of creatinine is roughly equivalent to 20 g of protein. *Thus, urinary creatinine serves as an index of lean body mass and can be used to assess muscle loss as follows:*

The patient's 24-hour urinary creatinine is measured and then compared to the ideal urinary creatinine found in normal persons (at their ideal weight) who are of the same sex, height, and body frame.[29-31] There should be some dietary control on the subjects to be tested since creatinine excretion is influenced by the ingestion of exogenous, preformed creatinine found in muscle protein

Table 8. MIDARM MUSCLE CIRCUMFERENCE (cm), Males*

Age (years)	Percentile						
	90th	75th	50th	25th	15th	10th	5th
18–24	30.8	28.9	27.2	25.8	25.0	24.4	23.5
25–34	31.7	30.0	28.0	26.5	25.8	25.3	24.2
35–44	32.1	30.3	28.7	27.1	26.2	25.6	25.0
45–54	31.5	29.8	28.1	26.5	25.6	24.9	24.0
55–64	31.0	29.6	27.9	26.2	25.4	24.4	22.8
65–74	29.9	28.5	26.9	25.3	24.3	23.7	22.5

MIDARM MUSCLE CIRCUMFERENCE (cm), Females*

Age (years)	Percentile						
	90th	75th	50th	25th	15th	10th	5th
18–24	23.6	22.1	20.6	19.4	18.8	18.5	17.7
25–34	24.9	22.9	21.4	20.0	19.3	18.9	18.3
35–44	26.1	24.0	22.0	20.6	19.7	19.2	18.5
45–54	26.6	24.3	22.2	20.7	19.9	19.5	18.8
55–64	26.3	24.4	22.6	20.8	20.1	19.5	18.6
65–74	26.5	24.4	22.5	20.8	20.0	19.5	18.6

*Reported by Bishop, et al[23,24] from data collected during the Health and Nutritional Examination Survey (HANES) of 1971–1974.[22] Adapted from *Am J Clin Nutr* 34: 2530–2539, 1981, with permission.
The following standards apply for determining nutritional status:[25]
 <5th percentile = Depleted
 5–15th percentile = Marginally depleted
 15–85th percentile = Normal
 >85th percentile = Above normal

(meat). Two or three consecutive 24-hour collections of urine are recommended. Normal values for creatinine excretion are 20–26 mg/kg body weight per 24 hours in men and 14–22 mg/kg per 24 hours in women.[28,31,32] To calculate the percentage of deficit for CHI, the following equation is used and then results compared to the standards shown in Tables 9 and 10 (pp. 23, 24):[18]

$$\text{CHI} = \frac{\text{mg urinary creatinine/24 hrs (patient)}}{\text{mg urinary creatinine/24 hrs (control)}} \times 100,$$

where control = a normal person (at ideal body weight) of the same sex, height, and body frame as the patient.

Based on percentage of the creatinine-height index, the degree of somatic protein depletion can be classified as follows:[18,19,30–32]

Table 9. **EXPECTED 24-HOUR URINARY CREATININE EXCRETION FOR MEN**

HEIGHT		SMALL FRAME		MEDIUM FRAME		LARGE FRAME	
in.	cm.	Ideal Wt. (KG)	mg Creatinine per 24°	Ideal Wt. (KG)	mg Creatinine per 24°	Ideal Wt. (KG)	mg Creatinine per 24°
61	154.9	52.7	1212	56.1	1290	60.7	1396
62	157.5	54.1	1244	57.7	1327	62.0	1426
63	160	55.4	1274	59.1	1359	63.6	1463
64	162.5	56.8	1306	60.4	1389	65.2	1500
65	165.1	58.4	1343	62.0	1426	66.8	1536
66	167.6	60.2	1385	63.9	1470	68.9	1585
67	170.2	62.0	1426	65.9	1516	71.1	1635
68	172.7	63.9	1470	67.7	1557	72.9	1677
69	175.3	65.9	1516	69.5	1598	74.8	1720
70	177.8	67.7	1557	71.6	1647	76.8	1766
71	180.3	69.5	1599	73.6	1693	79.1	1819
72	182.9	71.4	1642	75.7	1741	81.1	1865
73	185.4	73.4	1688	77.7	1787	83.4	1918
74	187.9	75.2	1730	80.0	1846	85.7	1971
75	190.5	77.0	1771	82.3	1893	87.7	2017

See the Creatinine-Height Index, page 21. These standards are likely to overestimate protein depletion in elderly patients. Ideal body weights are taken from the 1959 Metropolitan Insurance Company standards.
The values for "ideal" creatinine excretion listed for **men** are determined from the product of the ideal body weight in kilograms × 23 mg creatinine.
Adapted from Blackburn GL, et al, JPEN 1: 11–22, 1977,[18] with permission.

90–100% = normal
80– 90% = marginal depletion
60– 80% = moderate depletion
<60% = severe depletion

Creatinine excretion is reduced in wasting diseases where muscle is used for energy, resulting in loss of lean body mass.[29-31] Creatinine excretion also is lowered in renal disease;[33] therefore, the glomerular filtration rate must be normal, otherwise the CHI will not be accurate.[27,30] There are other disadvantages to using creatinine excretion in nutritional assessment: (1) Reference creatinine excretion values may not apply to every person, (2) Aging as a factor is not included in the reference tables, and (3) Trauma and sepsis can increase creatinine excretion. **Note:** *The*

Evaluating Nutritional Needs

Table 10. EXPECTED 24-HOUR URINARY CREATININE EXCRETION FOR WOMEN

HEIGHT		SMALL FRAME		MEDIUM FRAME		LARGE FRAME	
in.	cm.	Ideal Weight	mg Creatinine per 24°	Ideal Weight	mg Creatinine per 24°	Ideal Weight	mg Creatinine per 24°
56	142.2	43.2	778	46.1	830	50.7	913
57	144.8	44.3	797	47.3	851	51.8	932
58	147.3	45.4	817	48.6	875	53.2	958
59	149.8	46.8	842	50.0	900	54.5	981
60	152.4	48.2	868	51.4	925	55.9	1006
61	154.9	49.5	891	52.7	949	57.3	1031
62	157.5	50.9	916	54.3	977	58.9	1060
63	160.0	52.3	941	55.9	1006	60.6	1091
64	162.5	53.9	970	57.9	1042	62.5	1125
65	165.1	55.7	1003	59.8	1076	64.3	1157
66	167.6	57.5	1035	61.6	1109	66.1	1190
67	170.2	59.3	1067	63.4	1141	67.9	1222
68	172.7	61.4	1105	65.2	1174	70.0	1260
69	175.2	63.2	1138	67.0	1206	72.0	1296
70	177.8	65.0	1170	68.9	1240	74.1	1334

See the Creatinine-Height Index, page 21. These standards are likely to overestimate protein depletion in elderly patients. Ideal body weights are taken from the 1959 Metropolitan Insurance Company standards.
The values for "ideal" creatinine excretion listed for **women** are determined from the product of the ideal body weight in kilograms × 23 mg creatinine.
Adapted from Blackburn GL, et al, JPEN 1: 11–22, 1977,[18] with permission.

reader is referred to Table 11, which summarizes the degrees of calorie malnutrition (adult marasmus) based on anthropometric findings.

PART II: LABORATORY TESTS (Table 2)

Visceral Protein Status *(see adult kwashiorkor, p. 117).* Serum albumin, total iron binding capacity, transferrin (the iron-binding protein), lymphocytes, and immune competence are indicators of the patient's visceral protein status (Table 12). Abnormally low values of these proteins, lymphopenia, and a loss of cellular immunity are found in patients with a depleted visceral protein pool—a situation which can have dire consequences! Unfortunately, rapid restoration of protein stores in the ICU setting is unlikely, even with adequate nutrition.

Table 11. DEGREE OF CALORIE MALNUTRITION
(Adult Marasmus)

TEST	DEGREE OF MALNUTRITION
(1) % IDEAL BODY WEIGHT % IBW = $\dfrac{\text{Current Wt}}{\text{Ideal Wt}} \times 100$	80–90% = mild 60–80% = moderate See Tables 3–5, <60% = severe for ideal body wt.
(2) % USUAL WEIGHT % UW = $\dfrac{\text{Current Wt}}{\text{Usual Wt}} \times 100$	85–95% = mild 75–85% = moderate <75% = severe
(3) TRICEPS SKINFOLD	*See Table 6:* 5–15th percentile = marginally depleted 5th percentile = depleted
(4) MIDARM CIRCUMFERENCE	*See Table 7:* 5–15th percentile = marginally depleted 5th percentile = depleted
(5) MIDARM MUSCLE CIRCUMFERENCE MAMC = MAC (cm) − [3.14 × TSF (cm)]	*See Table 8:* 5–15th percentile = marginally depleted 5th percentile = depleted
(6) CREATININE-HEIGHT INDEX CHI = $\dfrac{\text{mg Urinary Creat/24 hrs (patient)}}{\text{mg Urinary Creat/24 hrs (control)}}$	*See Tables 9 & 10:* 80–90% = mild 60–80% = moderate <60% = severe

NOTE: The above anthropometric measurements fall to abnormally low levels in calorie malnutrition, whereas laboratory values (Table 12, p. 26) are usually preserved until the percent of ideal body weight goes below 85%.

(1) Serum Albumin. In evaluating the patient's nutritional status, serum albumin concentration is a far more reliable and sensitive index of protein malnutrition than the serum total protein[29] and has a close correlation with the arm muscle circumference.[34,35] The half-life of serum albumin is 18–20 days;[36] however, a significant drop can occur in less than 7 days in patients who are under stress (hypermetabolic, catabolic state) and are receiving mainly dextrose for both fluid and nutritional replacement.[37] In fact, serum albumin can decline 1.0 to 1.5 g/dl within 3 to 5 days in critically ill, catabolic patients because of leakage of protein from blood vessels. This condition is referred to as acute kwashiorkor-

Table 12. DEGREE OF PROTEIN MALNUTRITION
(Adult Kwashiorkor-Like State)

TEST	DEGREE OF MALNUTRITION
(1) ALBUMIN	3.5–5.5 g/dl = normal
	2.8–3.5 g/dl = mild
	2.1–2.7 g/dl = moderate
	<2.1 g/dl = severe
(2) TOTAL IRON BINDING CAPACITY (TIBC)	300–420 mcg/dl = normal
	200–250 mcg/dl = mild
	150–200 mcg/dl = moderate
	<150 mcg/dl = severe
(3) TRANSFERRIN (TSF)	200–350 mg/dl = normal
	150–175 mg/dl = mild
Serum TSF (mg/dl) =	100–150 mg/dl = moderate
(0.68 × TIBC) + 21	<100 mg/dl = severe
(4) TOTAL LYMPHOCYTES	1200–1800/ul = mild
	800–1200/ul = moderate
	<800/ul = severe
(5) SKIN TESTING FOR ANERGY (*Candida, Tricophyton,* PPD, mumps, tetanus)	Anergy to any of three antigens is consistent with severe malnutrition.
STATE OF PROTEIN METABOLISM	Normal = zero:

Nitrogen (N) Balance = $\dfrac{\text{grams protein (intake)}}{6.25}$ − (UUN + 4)

UUN = 24-hour urinary urea nitrogen in grams,
+4 = N lost via stool, intestinal gas, skin, plus urinary non-urea nitrogen
6.25 = Standard factor to convert protein to nitrogen (protein is 16% N)
Note = One gram of N loss = 30–32 grams of lean body mass!

like hypoalbuminemia (p. 117).[38] Based on levels of serum albumin, the degree of protein malnutrition can be classified as follows:[18,19]

2.8–3.5 g/dl = mild malnutrition
2.1–2.7 g/dl = moderate malnutrition
<2.1 g/dl = severe malnutrition

Major causes of hypoalbuminemia are as follows: poor protein intake (e.g., a cancer patient on chemotherapy or radiation therapy), impaired digestion (enteropathies, pancreatic disease), nitrogen loss (burns, trauma, renal disease), inadequate synthesis (sepsis, cirrhosis), hypoadrenalism, and overhydration. Abnormally increased values are found only in dehydration.[32] One should keep in mind that any sudden change in serum albumin concentration generally reflects the patient's status of hydration.

(2) **Total Iron Binding Capacity (TIBC) and Transferrin.** TIBC and transferrin are sensitive indicators of the body's protein status; both are lowered in patients who are under catabolic stress with loss of protein stores. *TIBC* includes serum iron (which is bound to transferrin) and the remaining iron-binding capacity of transferrin. Using an absorption technique, normal values for TIBC in our laboratory range from 300 to 400 mcg/dl. TIBC values below 250 mcg/dl are highly suggestive of deficiencies in transferrin,[39] and below 200 mcg/dl are indicative of malnutrition with a depleted visceral protein compartment.

Transferrin is a beta-1 globulin,[40] formerly called siderophilin, which is essential for the transport of iron (Fe^{+++}) in the plasma to the bone marrow. Normally transferrin is about 30% saturated with ferric iron (serum iron) and has a biologic half-life of only 8–10 days.[41] Because of its shorter half-life, transferrin is a much earlier indicator of protein deficiency than albumin [39,42] and reflects acute changes in visceral protein status.[43]

A quick approximation of serum transferrin can be derived from the total iron-binding capacity (mcg/dl) using the formula below:[44]

Serum transferrin (mg/dl) = (0.68 × TIBC) + 21.

We favor this equation over others* since the results have proven to be closer to the measured values; nevertheless, laboratory confirmation of transferrin levels is recommended whenever possible for greater accuracy. Kernstine and coworkers[36] have pointed out that equations estimating serum transferrin tend to be more inaccurate when significant malnutrition is present.

Other equations: Serum transferrin (mg/dl) = TIBC/1.45;
Serum transferrin (mg/dl) = (0.8 × TIBC) − 43, or
Serum transferrin (mg/dl) = (0.87 × TIBC) + 10.

To measure the amount of transferrin in the serum, an antigen-antibody reaction may be employed utilizing nephelometry. The normal range in our laboratory is 200–350 mg/dl. In protein-deficient patients, the reduced levels of transferrin are useful in classifying the degree of malnutrition:[18,19]

150–175 mg/dl = mild malnutrition
100–150 mg/dl = moderate malnutrition
<100 mg/dl = severe malnutrition

In addition to protein malnutrition, decreases in transferrin occur in pernicious anemia (untreated), chronic infection, liver disease, and iron overload.[32,38] On the other hand, elevated values are seen in iron deficiency and chronic blood loss. Like serum albumin, serum transferrin can be readily influenced by hydration; and in malnutrition, reduced levels are restored with proper nutrition.[37]

(3) **Other Plasma Proteins.**[45–48] Sensitive and rapid responding determinants of visceral protein loss are thyroxine-binding prealbumin (PA) and retinol-binding protein (RBP), both of which have short half-lives of 2–3 days and ½ day respectively. Reportedly, PA-RBP complex has the highest sensitivity to dietary deprivation and refeeding, compared to serum albumin (low sensitivity) and transferrin (intermediate sensitivity). The normal range in adults for prealbumin is 20–50 mg/dl and for retinol-binding protein is 37±7 mcg/dl. Currently, serum albumin and serum transferrin concentrations are the standard measurements to assess visceral protein.

(4) **Total Lymphocyte Count (TLC).** The total number of white blood cells (WBC) and lymphocytes (TLC) are simple but important determinations (TLC = WBC × % lymphocytes/100), especially in immunosuppressed patients who cannot mount a sufficient number of white blood cells to fight infection. Significant protein-calorie malnutrition is associated with a depressed immune system and lowered lymphocyte counts.[27,37,49,50] Using TLC as a standard, the patient's nutritional status (visceral protein compartment) can be classified as follows:[18,19]

1200–1800/microliter = mild malnutrition
800–1200/microliter = moderate malnutrition
<800/microliter = severe malnutrition

Importantly, refeeding will restore the lymphocyte count (and immune function) if malnutrition *per se* is the cause of the lymphopenia.[49,50] Other causes of lymphopenia include immunosuppressive therapeutic agents, radiation, viral infections, glucocorticoids, several congenital immunodeficiency states, chronic right ventricular failure, and so forth. **Note:** T-lymphocyte helper-suppressor ratio inversion may be a more sensitive indicator of protein-anergy malnutrition. (Diongi R: Proc Nutr Soc 41:355–371, 1982).

(5) **Skin Testing for Anergy.** As stated, malnutrition with visceral protein loss can rapidly lead to impairment of the immune system. In addition to total lymphocyte counts, checking the patient for delayed cutaneous hypersensitivity is helpful in evaluating the integrity of the immune system. The following antigens may be employed: *Candida, tricophyton,* PPD, mumps skin test antigen (MSTA™), and tetanus toxoid fluid extract (diluted 1:10 to 1:100). A convenient option is to use a factory-prepared device for delayed hypersensitivity skin testing (MULTITEST® CMI™). Each disposable set has 7 antigens and 1 control that is delivered on the forearm by intradermal skin prick. Streptokinase-streptodornase (Varidase) is no longer available commercially. The skin test site is examined for a reaction (measured in millimeters) which normally appears within 24 to 48 hours. Usually cellular immunity remains intact until the serum albumin falls below 3.0 g/dl or the percent ideal body weight drops below 85%.[18,37] Absence of any response to the antigens is seen in severe malnutrition. At our center, a reduced response (usually in the 3–5 mm range) is felt to be consistent with mild to moderate malnutrition. In settings where malnutrition is cause of anergy, a negative skin test may revert to a positive reaction with realimentation.[29,50] Many other factors, including steroids and chemotherapy, will suppress reactions to any of the antigens, and must be taken into consideration when appraising the results of skin tests. On the other hand, histamine H_2 receptor antagonists (cimetidine, ranitidine) may cause a false positive reaction by augmenting T lymphocyte activity[51]

(6) **Nitrogen (N) Balance.**[11,27,36,52] Measurement of N balance is a useful tool, especially in checking on the effectiveness of nutritional therapy. In healthy adults, N balance is regulated around zero, even in persons who eat substantial quantities of meat. In hospitalized patients, a reasonably good estimate of the state of protein metabolism during starvation/infection/injury (Figure 6) can be

Evaluating Nutritional Needs

STARVATION VS INJURY
Nitrogen Dynamics

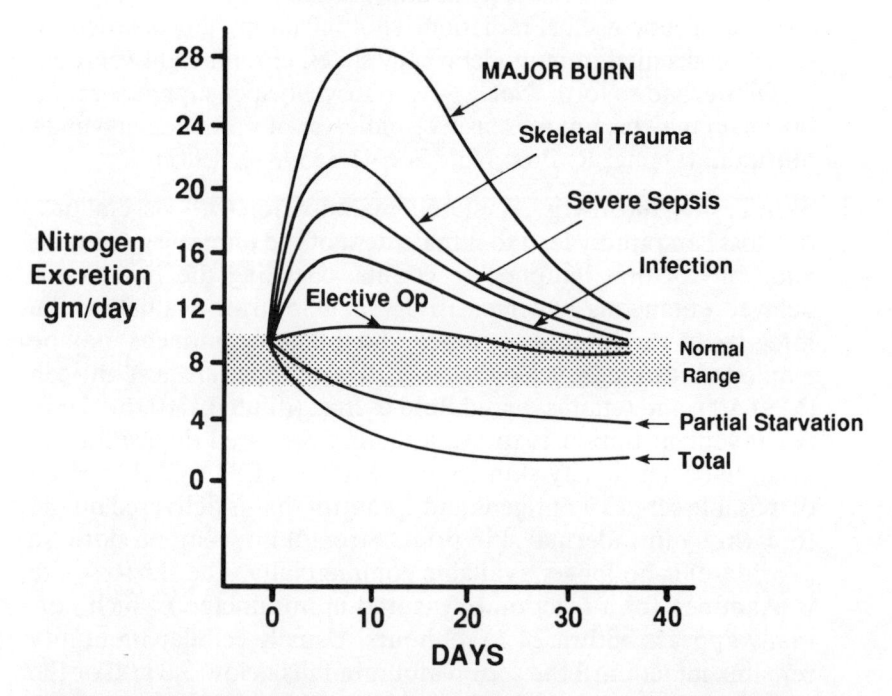

Figure 6. This illustration of urinary nitrogen excretion (g/day) demonstrates the increases which occur in hypermetabolic or **flow** states (burns, trauma, infection) and decreases in hypometabolic or **ebb** states (starvation, also shock). From Long CL, et al[7], with permission.

---

obtained by comparing the protein intake with nitrogen (N) loss in urine over a period of 24 hours. *The basic equation is:*

N balance = [N] intake − [N] output.

In the following calculation for nitrogen balance, bear in mind that approximately 90% of daily N loss is excreted via the urine* with 70–90% in the form of urea:[53,54]

$$\text{N balance} = \frac{\text{grams protein (intake)}}{6.25} - (\text{UUN} + 4), \text{ where}$$

UUN = 24-hour urinary urea nitrogen in grams,

---

*In chronic starvation or severe stress only 65% to 70% of N is excreted as UUN.[36]

+4 = N lost via stool, intestinal gas, skin, and urinary non-urea nitrogen (g/day),

6.25 = standard conversion factor that is used to change grams of protein into grams of nitrogen (protein is 16% nitrogen); for example, 100 grams PRO/6.25 = 16 grams N.

Example: A 55-year-old man with a 40% body-surface-area burn (wt. 80 kg, ht. 180 cm) has a daily protein intake of 50 grams and a urinary urea nitrogen loss of 19 grams/24 hours. Using the above formula for nitrogen balance, the daily N loss calculates to be -15 grams: $\frac{50}{6.25} - (19 + 4) = -15$ grams N/day. Since one gram of N loss = 30–32 grams of lean body mass,[55] the patient would lose 450–480 grams of muscle per day (subsequently visceral protein too), which is equivalent to at least one pound (450 grams = 1 lb)—a terrible price to pay! *If nitrogen loss continues uncorrected, then the potential consequences are delayed wound healing, infection, immunosuppression, muscle wasting, failure to thrive, organ failure, and ultimately death.* The desired goal in this patient (or in any instance where significant N loss exists) is to achieve a nitrogen balance of +1 to +4 in order to correct the deficit. The administration of 160 grams of PRO/day would give the patient a calculated positive N balance of 2.6 grams/day if his losses stay constant. N balance should be rechecked throughout the patient's illness since protein requirements decrease with healing.

Comments: The above standard formula for nitrogen balance does not take into account N losses due to nasoenteric tube suction, malabsorption, enteropathy, enterocutaneous fistula, desquamative disease, kidney failure, or liver failure. In fact, severely stressed, catabolic patients may have large enough losses of nonurea nitrogen to cause them to be in negative nitrogen balance while the formula spuriously indicates a positive balance. For example, excessive amino acid losses in the urine may require measurement of total urinary nitrogen (TUN) or simply estimating the TUN by the following modified formula:[36]

[N] excreted = 1–2 g (skin, stool),
+ UUN (g),
+ (0.10–0.35) × UUN (g).

In the uremic patient, an adjustment is made in calculating N balance by adding the change in blood urea nitrogen to the total urinary nitrogen (or UUN + 4) as follows:[19]

TUN (or UUN + 4) + [Bun$_f$ − BUN$_i$) × (0.6 W)] + [W$_f$ − W$_i$) × BUN$_f$],
where TUN = total urinary nitrogen (g/day), f = final, i = initial, BUN = blood urea nitrogen (g/l), W = body weight in kg, and 0.6 = the fraction of body weight that is water.

This modified equation is applicable to measurements taken over 1–3 days and also can be used in hemodialysis patients during the intervals between dialysis. The measurements, however, do not apply to peritoneal dialysis patients because of protein lost in the dialysate.

Note: *The reader is referred to Table 12, which summarizes the degrees of protein malnutrition (adult kwashiorkor), based on laboratory findings.*

OTHER IMPORTANT LABORATORY TESTS

Serum Phosphorus. The element phosphorus is the main intracellular anion in the body. Normal levels of serum phosphorus range from 2.5 mg/dl to 4.5 mg/dl, but values may fall rapidly in stressful situations (during the anabolic phase of nutritional repletion) if increased requirements for phosphorus are not met.[56] Patients on respirators or patients recovering from burns, being tube fed, receiving phosphate-binding antacids, or being administered feedings high in CHO should routinely be checked for hypophosphatemia.[57,58] *A serum value between 1.0 and 2.5 mg/dl is indicative of moderate hypophosphatemia and if lower than 1.0 mg/dl is diagnostic of severe hypophosphatemia.* Harmful physiological effects include a decrease in 2,3 diphosphoglycerate (DPG), a shift to the left in the oxyhemoglobin dissociation curve, reduced O_2 transport,[59] and a decrease in tissue adenosine triphosphate (ATP).[57] Clinically, patients with low serum levels of phosphorus (below 1.5 to 1.0 mg/dl) may demonstrate mental confusion, seizures, muscular weakness (skeletal myopathy), hemolytic anemia, cardiac failure (cardiomyopathy), arrhythmias, decreased tissue sensitivity to insulin, abnormal calcium and magnesium metabolism, and respiratory failure.[57,60–63] The recommended dietary allowance for adults is 800 mg/day (National Research Council, 1980). During TPN (amino acids + dextrose + lipid emulsions + additives), the usual maintenance dose of phosphorus is about 40–60 mEq/day (30–40 mM/day of sodium or potassium phosphate; see p. 124). Another source of phosphorus comes from the phospholipids in fat emulsion.[64] **Note:** In renal failure, phosphate is removed from TPN solutions.

Serum Magnesium. The element magnesium is a rather abundant cation in the body and is intimately involved in cellular metabolism and oxidative phosphorylation. Magnesium (Mg) is distributed chiefly as an intracellular and skeletal ion (free form) with less than 1% being extracellular. In general, serum magnesium levels in the range of 1.2–1.8 mg/dl are classified as mild hypomagnesemia and below 1.0 mg/dl as severe hypomagnesemia. Clinically, low levels of Mg frequently are seen in bowel disorders (malabsorption, extensive small bowel resection), acute pancreatitis, and Mg-wasting renal diseases. A number of clinical syndromes have been attributed to severe hypomagnesemia (≤ 1 mg/dl), which primarily involve the neuromuscular, cardiovascular, and gastrointestinal systems. However, many of these patients also have concomitant hypokalemia and/or hypocalcemia, making it difficult to separate one deficiency from the other.* In addition, there often is *poor correlation* between the level of total serum Mg (which includes ionized, chelated, and protein-bound fractions) and clinical signs or symptoms.[65] *In fact, many patients with low serum Mg remain asymptomatic!* Zaloga also points out that currently there is no one laboratory test that unerringly reveals Mg deficiency and that free intracellular Mg may prove to be a better indicator of Mg deficiency. Unfortunately, the technique for this measurement is not yet readily available.

Although there is no single test that serves as a completely reliable indicator of Mg deficiency, one useful option (used in the pediatric age group) is to carry out a Mg load test with measured urinary recovery.[66] For accurate results, the patient must not have kidney dysfunction or a renal tubular wasting syndrome. Under these conditions, minimal loss of magnesium equates with renal conservation in the presence of a deficiency state.

In spite of the aforesaid comments, a common clinical practice is to replace magnesium in patients who are receiving TPN, utilizing a dosage of 8–10 mEq/day. But in profound magnesium wasting syndromes, intakes as high as 40–60 mEq/day may be necessary. Following IV administration, Mg levels should be checked right away and repeated 4–6 hours later to make certain that replacement has been

---

*In some instances, it is not possible to correct hypokalemia or hypocalcemia until magnesium stores are repleted.

adequate. In patients who have renal failure with little or no urinary output, one must be cautious giving Mg.

Miscellaneous. In the absence of liver disease, a *serum cholesterol* level below 150 mg/dl is commonly seen in malnutrition. A low *blood urea nitrogen* (normal range 10–20 mg/dl) suggests the possibility of inadequate intake of protein. A deficiency in *zinc* (cofactor for many enzymes) often occurs in patients with protein malnutrition. Another cofactor for numerous enzymes, *serum magnesium* (see above), often has values below 1.5 mEq/L in chronic malnutrition.

Note: The reader is referred to the discussion on sodium chloride, potassium, and calcium on pages 89, 90. Also information regarding minerals and trace metals is located on page 99. **For a thorough review of the administration of essential vitamins and trace elements (including macrominerals and microminerals) the reader is referred to four excellent sources:**

(1) Baumgartner TB (ed): *Clinical Guide to Parenteral Micronutrition,* 1st edition, Melrose Park, IL, Educational Publications, LTD, 1984.

(2) Bernard MA, Jacobs, DO, Rombeau JL: *Nutrition and Metabolic Support of Hospitalized Patients,* Philadelphia, WB Saunders Co, 1986.

(3) Halpern SL (ed): *Quick Reference to Clinical Nutrition,* Philadelphia, Lea & Febiger, 1987.

(4) Tuckerman MM, Turco SJ (eds): *Human Nutrition,* Philadelphia, Lea & Febiger, 1983.

CHAPTER 3
EVALUATING NUTRITIONAL NEEDS

PART III: PREDICTION EQUATIONS FOR ENERGY REQUIREMENTS

Prediction formulas **estimate** the resting energy expenditure (REE) and should serve only as guidelines in patient management. Foster and coworkers[16] recently carried out a landmark study in which 100 TPN patients were measured by indirect calorimetry and the results cross-matched with 191 different prediction equations. *This study proved that predictions, when compared to the accuracy of indirect calorimetry, are **not** as reliable in determining the energy needs of most patients.* Our findings here support Foster's work, especially in critical care situations. Nevertheless, the following equations have played an important role in the nutritional assessment of the ill or traumatized patient, and some are still being used.

(1) Long's Calculations, Based Solely on Body Weight[6]

Condition	kcal/kg/day
Healthy:	
resting	23–24
light activity	28–29
Skeletal trauma	28–30
Sepsis	35
3rd ° burn	45
(>60% BSA)	

Note: The above values are the estimated energy requirements for *resting* metabolism. *Activity* increases caloric requirements by approximately 20%. Predictions based only on kcal/kg are the least accurate way of estimating caloric needs!

Evaluating Nutritional Needs

(2) The Quebbeman-Ausman Regression Equation[67]

FOR MALES: REE (kcal/24 hrs) = W × 12.3 + 754,

FOR FEMALES: REE (kcal/24 hrs) = W × 6.9 + 879,
where W = weight in kg.

Note: The result obtained is multiplied by an activity factor of 1.2 for total energy expenditure (kilocalories/day).

(3) Regression Equation Based on Body Surface Area[67]

FOR MALES: REE (kcal/24 hrs) = BSA × 789 + 137,

FOR FEMALES: REE (kcal/24 hrs) = BSA × 544 + 414,
where BSA = body surface area in square meters:[10]
BSA = $W^{0.425}$ × $H^{0.725}$ × .007184 (W = weight in kg; H = height in cm)

(4) The Krause-Mahan Calculations for Total Energy Expenditure (TEE)[5]

(a) First, determine the ideal body weight (IBW) as shown in Tables 3 and 4, or 5.

(b) Next, calculate the daily basal needs. FOR MEN: 1.0 kcal × IBW [kg] × 24 hours. FOR WOMEN: 0.95 × kcal × IBW [kg] × 24 hours.

(c) Then, subtract 0.1 kcal × IBW [kg] × hours of sleep.

(d) Add an activity increment of 30%, 50%, 75%, or 100%.

(e) Finally, add 10% above the energy requirement to account for the specific dynamic action (SDA) of food.

EXAMPLE:
The subject is a 55-year-old male who has a height of 180 cm, weight 80 kg, and a medium frame.

IBW (Table 5)	= 47 kg + [(180 − 152/2.54 cm) × (2.2 kg)] = 71 kg,
Basal needs	= 1.0 kcal × 71 kg × 24 hrs = 1704 kcal,
Sleep	= 0.1 kcal × 71 kg × 8 hrs = 57 kcal, 1704 − 57 = 1647 kcal.
Activity (light)	= 50% above basal = 852 kcal, 1647 + 852 = 2499 kcal.

SDA (specific
dynamic action) = 10% above energy requirement = 250 kcal,

TEE = 2499 + 250 = 2749 kcal/day.

(5) The Harris-Benedict Equation[68]

This well-known calculation estimates the resting energy expenditure (REE) in kilocalories over a 24-hour period. The equation is largely dependent on body weight and is *unreliable* in situations where the patient's metabolism has been altered by disease, trauma, thermal injury, surgery, infection, sepsis, or chemotherapy.[1,16,69] In spite of these inherent problems, the Harris-Benedict equation, introduced 70 years ago, is still widely employed. Once having calculated the subject's total daily energy need, the value obtained (REE) is empirically multiplied by a *stress factor* and also an *activity factor* as shown below:[70]

**TOTAL CALORIES NEEDED* =
RESTING ENERGY EXPENDITURE (REE)
× ACTIVITY FACTOR × STRESS FACTOR:**

REE FOR MALES (kcal/24 hrs) = [66.473 + (13.752 × W) + (5.003 × H)] − (6.755 × A);

REE FOR FEMALES (kcal/24 hrs) = [655.096 + (9.563 × W) + (1.85 × H)] − (4.676 × A);

where W = weight in kg, H = height in cm, and A = age in years.

ACTIVITY FACTOR: confined to bed = 1.2
out of bed = 1.3

STRESS FACTOR:

minor surgery	= 1.1	skeletal trauma	= 1.35
major surgery	= 1.2	blunt trauma	= 1.35
mild infection	= 1.2	head injury + steroids	= 1.6
modt. infection	= 1.4	40% body area burn	= 1.5
severe infection	= 1.8	100% body area burn	= 2.0

*A quick method to approximate protein requirements is to multiply the *total calories needed* by the *factor 0.0416* (Ross Laboratories, Columbus, OH).

Evaluating Nutritional Needs

Note: For comparison, see Table 13 (p. 39) for stress factors listed by Cerra.[71]

EXAMPLE:
The patient is a 55-year-old male with moderately severe COPD and bilateral pneumonia who has been on a mechanical ventilator for 3 days. He is being given IV 5% dextrose + half-normal saline to meet his fluid requirements. Renal function is normal. Therapy consists of oxygen (FIO_2 0.4), antibiotics, and bronchodilators. He has shown some improvement but definitely is not yet a candidate for weaning from the ventilator. His weight is 80 kg and height 180 cm. Using the Harris-Benedict equation:

TOTAL ENERGY NEED/24 hrs = REE × ACTIVITY FACTOR × STRESS FACTOR =

[66.47 + (13.75 × 80) + (5 × 180)] − (6.76 × 55) =

$\underset{\text{(REE)}}{1695} \times \underset{\text{(ACTIVITY)}}{1.2} \times \underset{\text{(STRESS)}}{1.3}$ = 2847 kcal / 24 hrs.

Question: Are the above factors correct for activity and stress? Can one be certain that the patient's calculated energy requirement is 2847 kcal / day?

Answer: Indirect calorimetry is necessary to accurately measure the total amount of energy (kcal / day) needed by the patient and to obtain an RQ to assess the substrate mixture! The goal here is to avoid overfeeding, underfeeding, or excessive carbohydrate while maintaining adequate protein and fat.

(6) The Moore-Angelillo Equation[72]
This selective equation is used to predict the resting energy expenditure over a 24-hour period in ambulatory patients with moderate to severe COPD:

FOR MALES: REE (kilocalories/24 hours) = (11.5 × W) + 952;

FOR FEMALES: REE (kilocalories/24 hours) = (14.1 × W) + 515;

Where W = weight in kg.

Table 13. LEVELS OF STRESS AND NUTRITIONAL NEEDS*

Stress Level	Clinical Situation	Total Stress Factor (× REE)	Total Urinary N Loss (g/day)	Protein (amino acids, g/kg/day)	NPC:N	Total Calories (kcal/kg/day)
0	Simple starvation	1.0	<5	1.0	150:1	28
1	General surgery	1.2–1.3	5–10	1.5	100:1	32
2	Multiple trauma	1.3–1.5	10–15	1.5–2.0	100:1	32–40
3	Sepsis (early)	1.5	15–20	2.0	80:1	40
4	Sepsis (late); Severe burns	2.0	>20	2.5	80:1	50

NOTE: NPC:N = non-protein calories to grams of nitrogen ratio.
Patients at stress level 1 are anabolic and at level 2 may be mildly catabolic.
Patients at stress levels 3 and 4 have significant catabolic metabolism, hence the need for restoration of lean body mass. COPD patients on ventilators often have a stress factor of around 1.3. This value is higher if they are septic.

*Adapted from Cerra F: Pocket Manual of Surgical Nutrition, St. Louis, The Mosby Co., 1984, p. 60, with permission.

EXAMPLE:

The patient is a 55-year-old male who has the same body measurements as the patient above and also has moderate to moderately severe COPD. The only differences are that he is ambulatory and does not have pneumonia. Using the Moore-Angelillo equation, his 24-hour REE is calculated as follows:

REE = (11.5 × 80) + 952 = 1872 kcal per day.

(7) The Curreri Formula[73] and Other Prediction Guidelines[74]

The Curreri equation was especially designed to help estimate nutritional needs for *burn* patients:

CEE (kcal/24 hrs) = [(25 × W) + % BSA burned)], where
    CEE = Curreri energy expenditure,
    W = body weight in kg,
    BSA = body surface area. The Rule of Nines may be used to estimate the percentage of burned surface area.

Evaluating Nutritional Needs

The Rule of Nines. For initial assessment of the burned area in an adult or a child, the Rule of Nines may be employed:

Adult Body Part	% of Total Body Surface	Child Body Part	% of Total Body Surface
Arm (shoulder to fingertips)	9%	Arm (shoulder to fingertips)	9%
Head and Neck	9%	Head and Neck	18%
Leg (groin to toe)	18%	Anterior Trunk	18%
Anterior Trunk	18%	Posterior Trunk	18%
Posterior Trunk	18%	Leg (groin to toe)	14%
Perineum	1%		

Greater accuracy in calculating body surface area may be achieved (especially in children) by using a modified Lund-Browder Chart that is based on the patient's age.[75,76]

Comment: Our experience has been that the Curreri formula tends to overestimate the average daily energy needs of burn patients over the course of their illness by as much as 10–15%. Therefore, prior to acquiring a metabolic cart, we used the Harris-Benedict formula multiplied by a factor of 1.2 to 2.0 (sliding scale) depending upon the percentage of burned surface area and the stage of the injury (acute/intermediate/late period):

ACUTE THERMAL INJURY

Body Surface Burned	Correction Factor
0–20%	1.0–1.5
20–40%	1.5–1.85
40–100%	1.85–2.05

Other guidelines (not precise) for burn patients are the following energy and protein requirements:[74]

ENERGY REQUIREMENTS IN BURNS
(Cal/m²/24 hr)

	0–40% Burn	>40% Burn
Child 6–10 yrs	1350–1450	1950–2050
Adolescent	1200–1300	1675–1750
Young Adult	1100–1150	1550–1625

PROTEIN REQUIREMENTS FOR EQUILIBRIUM IN BURNS

Period	Postburn Day	Protein Requirements (g/kg body weight/day)	
1	7–16	3.20–3.94	Catabolic phase (Average N balance is −4.5 g/day)
2	30–39	2.02–2.53	
3	60–69	1.44–0.51	
4	90–99	1.08–0.51	

Note: The caloric cost of insensible water loss from *intact skin* is about 600 Cal/m²/day (about 21% of daily heat loss). In burn patients, until grafting is complete, there is tremendous water evaporation from the denuded, raw surface, presenting additional problems in adjusting fluid balance and caloric requirements. In fact, it is not unusual for a severe burn patient to lose 4 L of fluid/day, which is equivalent to approximately 2000 kcal/day needed as a result of the water loss alone.[6,27] *The **bottom line** is that indirect calorimetry is necessary to accurately follow the rapidly changing energy requirements in acutely burned patients, thus avoiding undernutrition or overnutrition.* See page 76 for information on feeding burn patients.

PART IV: INDIRECT CALORIMETRY
Introduction

The most accurate way to evaluate the patient's nutritional needs is by indirect calorimetry.[1,16,69] Using a computerized metabolic cart, the

Evaluating Nutritional Needs

energy requirements of the patient can be determined on the basis of oxygen consumption ($\dot{V}O_2$), carbon dioxide production ($\dot{V}CO_2$), and urinary nitrogen (see Weir's equation below).[1,77-83] For resolving substrate utilization, the ratio of the $\dot{V}CO_2$ to the $\dot{V}O_2$ (respiratory quotient or RQ) can be easily calculated—something not possible using prediction equations. Armed with accurate gas exchange data, anthropometrics and laboratory results, one can avoid many of the feeding problems often encountered in critically ill patients, such as overfeeding or underfeeding patients with lung disease, trauma, sepsis, thermal injury, and so on. In addition to ascertaining that the correct number of calories and grams of protein (PRO) are begin given, adjustments can be made in the substrate (CHO, FAT) to achieve an ideal RQ between 0.8 to 0.85.

Calculations Based on Indirect Calorimetry

(1) **Weir's Equation.** This formula was published in 1949 by Weir[83] and is the accepted "standard" to calculate the resting energy expenditure.

REE (kcal / 24 hrs) =
$$[3.941\,(\dot{V}O_2) + 1.106\,(\dot{V}CO_2)]\,1.44 - (2.17\,UN), \text{where}$$

REE = resting energy expenditure in kilocalories/day
$\dot{V}O_2$ = oxygen uptake in ml/min
$\dot{V}CO_2$ = carbon dioxide production in ml/min
UN = total urinary nitrogen in grams/day (urea + nonurea nitrogen)
$1.44 = \dfrac{1440\,(min/day)}{1000\,(ml/liter)}$

(2) **Weir's Abbreviated Equation.** Instead of using the complete Weir equation (which requires a 24-hour collection of urine for UN), one can conveniently utilize the following shortened form and still obtain values that are *within 2% of the original formula:*[84]

REE (kcal / 24 hrs) = $[3.9\,(\dot{V}O_2) + 1.1\,(\dot{V}CO_2)]\,1.44$ (See p. 63 for an example)

Note: Based on the work of Swinamer et al,[85] the value obtained by either of Weir's equations shown above should be multiplied by an **"activity" factor** of 1.10. This 10% upward adjustment is to allow for the various routine, daily activities involving the patient in the intensive care unit (ICU).

(3) Shortcut Equation. One can use the following elementary formula to quickly approximate the resting energy expenditure:

REE (kcal/24 hrs) = $\dot{V}O_2$ L/24 hrs × 5 or

REE (kcal/24 hrs) = $\dot{V}O_2$ ml/min (mean value) × 7.2

This calculation, however, is correct only when the RQ ($\dot{V}CO_2/\dot{V}O_2$) is 1.0. Actually, the caloric value of oxygen is dependent upon the type of nutrient being oxidized. Since O_2 Caloric Value = (1.23 × $\dot{V}CO_2/\dot{V}O_2$) + 3.81, the energy production of oxygen is shown below as a function of RQ for a carbohydrate-fat mixture:

RQ ($\dot{V}CO_2/\dot{V}O_2$)	O_2 Caloric Value
1.0	5.04
0.90	4.92
0.80	4.79
0.71	4.68

Note: Commonly used equations to estimate or measure REE are summarized in Table 14, page 44.

Calorimetry at the Bedside

Old methods of measuring gas exchange by the Tissot spirometer or Douglas bag collections of expired air were laborious and time consuming. Currently, metabolic assessment for energy needs is tremendously facilitated by indirect calorimetry whereby one can utilize a metabolic cart to carry out measurements at the patient's bedside either on the ward, burn unit, or in the ICU (Figure 7). *To collect accurate data, it is vitally important that proper technique be employed.*

(1) Measurement Conditions (general rules)

   (a) **The patient must rest quietly** for at least 30 minutes prior to testing and have no food or drink for the previous 2 hours (see *item g* for the exception). Significant increases in body metabolism may be caused by any stimulation of the patient, for example, suctioning, repositioning, bathing, feeding, chest physical therapy, and visitation by relatives or friends (Figure 9). Hannenberg and colleagues[86] recommended that one hour elapse while the patient's temperature, level of awareness, and body metabolism remain stabilized.

Evaluating Nutritional Needs

Table 14. EQUATIONS FOR RESTING ENERGY EXPENDITURE

THE HARRIS-BENEDICT EQUATION (to estimate REE):

FOR MALES: REE (kcal/24 hrs) = [66.473 + (13.752 × W) + (5.003 × H)] − (6.755 × A)

FOR FEMALES: REE (kcal/24 hrs) = [655.096 + (9.563 × W) + (1.85 × H)] − (4.676 × A)

REE = resting energy expenditure
W = weight in kg
H = height in cm
A = age in years

WEIR'S EQUATION (to measure REE):

REE (kcals/24 hrs) = [3.941 ($\dot{V}O_2$) + 1.106 ($\dot{V}CO_2$)] 1.44 − (2.17 UN)

WEIR'S ABBREVIATED EQUATION:

REE (kcals/24 hrs) = [3.9 ($\dot{V}O_2$) + 1.1 ($\dot{V}CO_2$)] 1.44

$\dot{V}O_2$ = oxygen uptake in ml/min
$\dot{V}CO_2$ = carbon dioxide produced in ml/min
UN = total urinary nitrogen (N) in grams/day

1.44 = $\dfrac{1440 \text{ (min/day)}}{1000 \text{ (ml/liter)}}$

SHORTCUT EQUATIONS:

REE (kcal/24 hrs) = $\dot{V}O_2$L/24 hrs × 5, or
 = $\dot{V}O_2$ml/min × 7.2

NOTE: O_2 Caloric Value = (1.23 × $\dot{V}CO_2/\dot{V}O_2$) + 3.81

Evaluating Nutritional Needs

(b) **The environment** should be as quiet and comfortable as possible with a stable room temperature, ideally 21° to 23° C.

(c) **The patient should not be permitted to go to sleep** during the test.

(d) **For patients on ventilators,** any of the ventilatory variables (rate of breathing, tidal volume, etc.) should not be altered for at least 90 minutes prior to measuring $\dot{V}O_2$ and $\dot{V}CO_2$ in order to achieve a steady level of gas exchange.

(e) **If the patient is being mechanically ventilated,** then adjustments must be made for airflow and for any supplemental oxygen being administered. The FIO_2 being delivered to the patient must be reasonably stable, delivered uniformly through the inspiratory line (a nasal cannula cannot be used), and accurately measured. *At FIO_2 values above 0.5–0.6, inaccuracies occur that render the test invalid.*[85,87]

(f) **The one-minute data points** obtained for $\dot{V}O_2$ and $\dot{V}CO_2$ should not vary from their mean values for the test period by more than ±5%.

(g) **If nutrients are being given continuously** by enteral or parenteral route, then the rate of infusion must be steady while testing is carried out.

(h) **For metabolically stable patients:** All of the data used to derive the REE and RQ must be taken while the patient is in a "steady state" (see *item a* above) and collected over a 30-minute period.[88] Some operators have extended the testing period to as long as 45 to 60 minutes.[89,90] But an average time of 20–30 minutes, repeated 2 to 4 times daily, has proven to be satisfactory at our medical center, providing the patient is stable.

(i) **For metabolically unstable patients:** Intermittent or "window" studies may not be adequate for unstable, critically ill patients who have fluctuating metabolic rates (e.g., septic or burn patients). These individuals require *continuous* metabolic monitoring of 16–24 hours (a minimum of 8 hours in some instances) to obtain accurate data reflecting the patient's true, overall status. *In the near future, computerized metabolic monitors used in intensive care situations will be integrated*

Evaluating Nutritional Needs

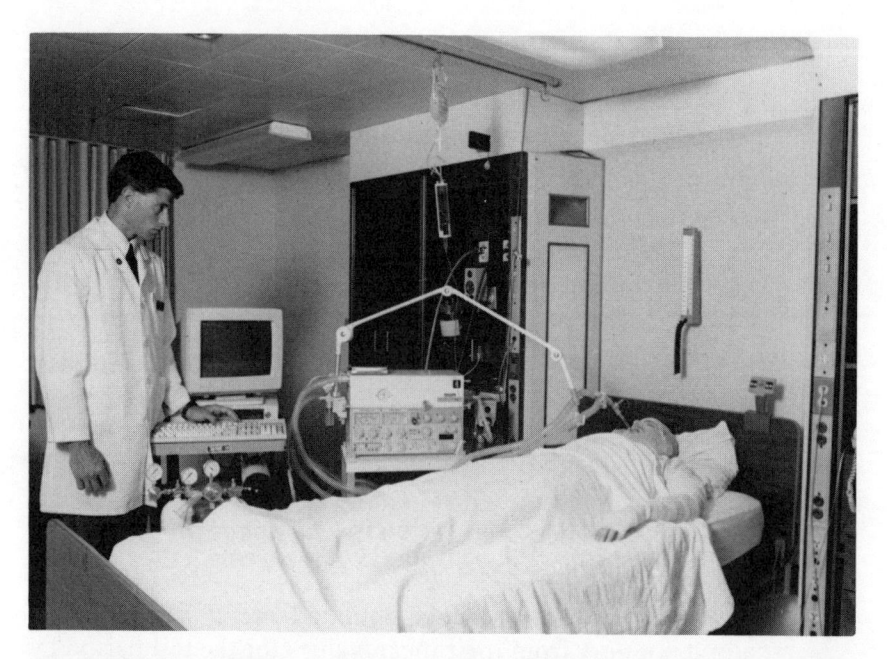

Figure 7. **The Medical Graphics CCM (Critical Care Monitor)** is shown measuring REE on a mechanically ventilated patient who sustained extensive burns and smoke inhalation, complicated by pneumonia. Subsequently, successful weaning from the Servo Ventilator 900 C (Siemans Elma, Sweden) was carried out.

with ventilators as single units (for continuous monitoring) rather than functioning as separate, free-standing systems.

(j) **Regarding equipment for measuring REE,** there are advantages to using a breath-by-breath analyzer rather than a mixing-type of chamber (page 56, *item 5*). On nonventilator patients, increased accuracy and reliability can be achieved by utilizing a new accessory device known as Medical Graphic's hood or "bubble" (Figures 8a, 8b) that fits over the patient's head and has an internal funnel located directly in front of the mouth to sample each breath. Also MGC's Desktop CCM (Medical Graphic Corporation's Critical Care Monitor) has a unique, useful feature whereby any inadvertent or unexpected burst of excessive metabolic activity (reflected by a sudden surge of high $\dot{V}O_2$ and CO_2 values on the CRT screen) can be selectively eliminated from the baseline values at the end of a test run (Figure 9).

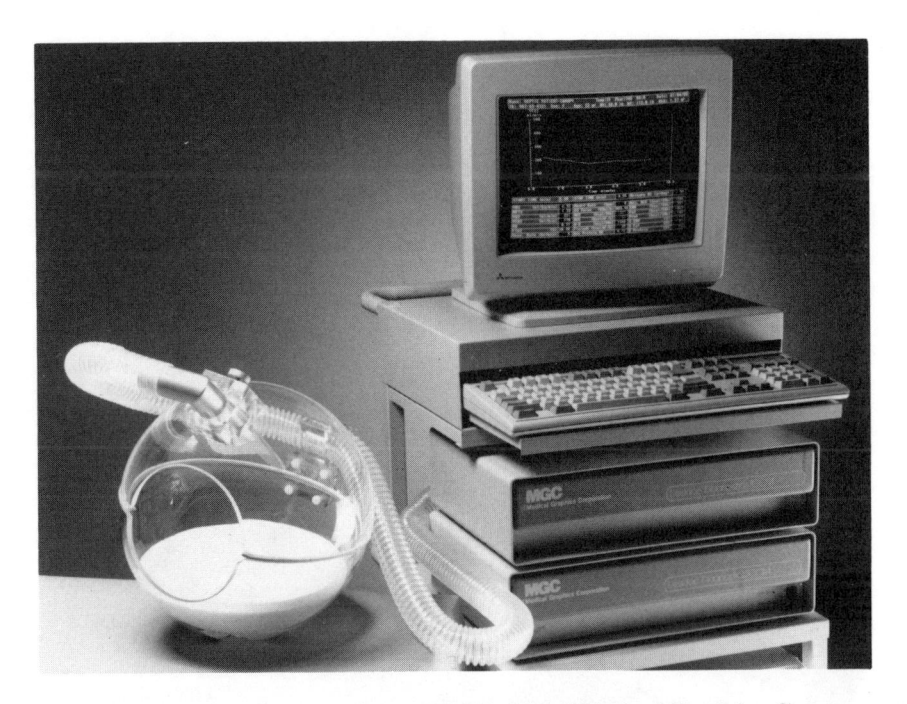

Figure 8a. A close-up view of the **MGC Bubble (Medical Graphics Corporation).** The unique feature of this type of hood is the capacity for breath-by-breath analysis rather than having the apparatus function as a mixing chamber. Interestingly, equilibrium is reached after only 2–3 breaths.

(2) **Operation and Quality Control.** The manufacturers and distributors of critical care metabolic monitors have their own instructions on how to operate the equipment. Much of the methodology is similar; however, one should *carefully review the user's manual.* A warm-up time of one hour is usually required prior to calibration of the pneumotachometer and gas analyzers. The pneumotachometer is standardized with a 3.0 liter super-syringe, at slow, moderate, and fast rates. The O_2 and CO_2 gas analyzers are carefully adjusted with known concentrations of dry gas, namely, 14% to 17% O_2 and 5% to 7% CO_2. Ambient room temperature (degrees Celsius), barometric pressure (millimeters of mercury), relative humidity (in percent), and valve dead space (60–100 ml) are entered into the computer during the calibration routine. For systems employing breath-by-breath analysis, the response time of the O_2 and CO_2 analyzers must be determined and the phase delay (between the flow signal and gas signals) closely checked and

Evaluating Nutritional Needs

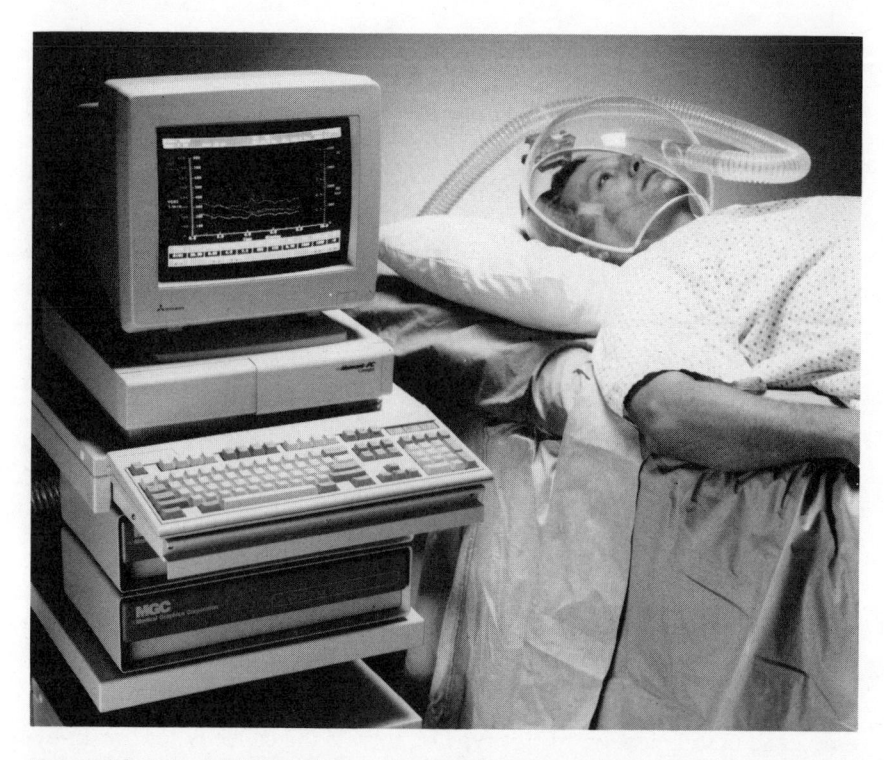

Figure 8b. **The MGC Bubble** is shown with the patient's head resting comfortably inside the transparent, plastic cover. Data from each breath of the spontaneously breathing subject is recorded on the CRT screen.

aligned. **Note:** Information on the basic physiologic principles of indirect calorimetry (including determinations, calculations, etc.) is available in Zavala's handbook titled *"Manual On Exercise Testing",* Publication Order Service, Oakdale Hall, The University of Iowa, Iowa City, Iowa 52242.

(3) **Equipment.** With the exception of Engstrom, the manufacturers listed below all make and distribute metabolic carts in the United States for measuring REE on both spontaneously breathing and mechanically ventilated patients. Engstrom has built their metabolic unit (computer, O_2 analyzer, CO_2 analyzer, pneumotachometer) as an attachable but integral part of the Engstrom Erica mechanical ventilator rather than as a separate, free-standing unit.

Evaluating Nutritional Needs

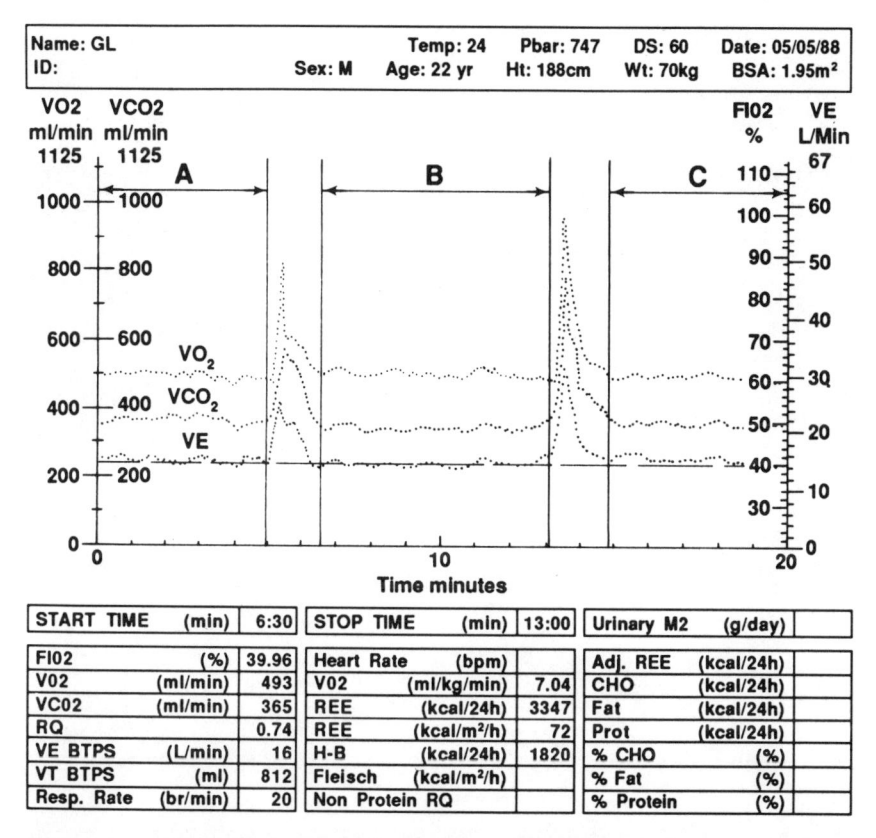

Name: GL		Temp: 24	Pbar: 747	DS: 60	Date: 05/05/88
ID:	Sex: M	Age: 22 yr	Ht: 188cm	Wt: 70kg	BSA: 1.95m²

START TIME	(min)	6:30	STOP TIME	(min)	13:00	Urinary M2	(g/day)	
FIO2	(%)	39.96	Heart Rate	(bpm)		Adj. REE	(kcal/24h)	
VO2	(ml/min)	493	VO2	(ml/kg/min)	7.04	CHO	(kcal/24h)	
VCO2	(ml/min)	365	REE	(kcal/24h)	3347	Fat	(kcal/24h)	
RQ		0.74	REE	(kcal/m²/h)	72	Prot	(kcal/24h)	
VE BTPS	(L/min)	16	H-B	(kcal/24h)	1820	% CHO	(%)	
VT BTPS	(ml)	812	Fleisch	(kcal/m²/h)		% Fat	(%)	
Resp. Rate	(br/min)	20	Non Protein RQ			% Protein	(%)	

Figure 9. A 20-minute metabolic run by indirect calorimetry on **Medical Graphics CCM** is shown above. This breath-by-breath measurement of REE (see Case Study, page 59), illustrates what can happen during periods of seemingly harmless stimulation. The first episode of hypermetabolism occurred when the patient's sister inadvertently began talking to him, and the second occurred when his wife entered the room! The two separate surges of high oxygen uptake ($\dot{V}O_2$), carbon dioxide production ($\dot{V}CO_2$), and minute ventilation ($\dot{V}_E$) were selectively removed, leaving the stable panels A, B, and C as representative of baseline resting values.

The major manufacturers of critical care monitors include:

Medical Graphics Corporation (Figure 10)
350 Oak Grove Parkway
St. Paul, MN 55127
Telephone 612/484–4874 or 1-800-333-4137

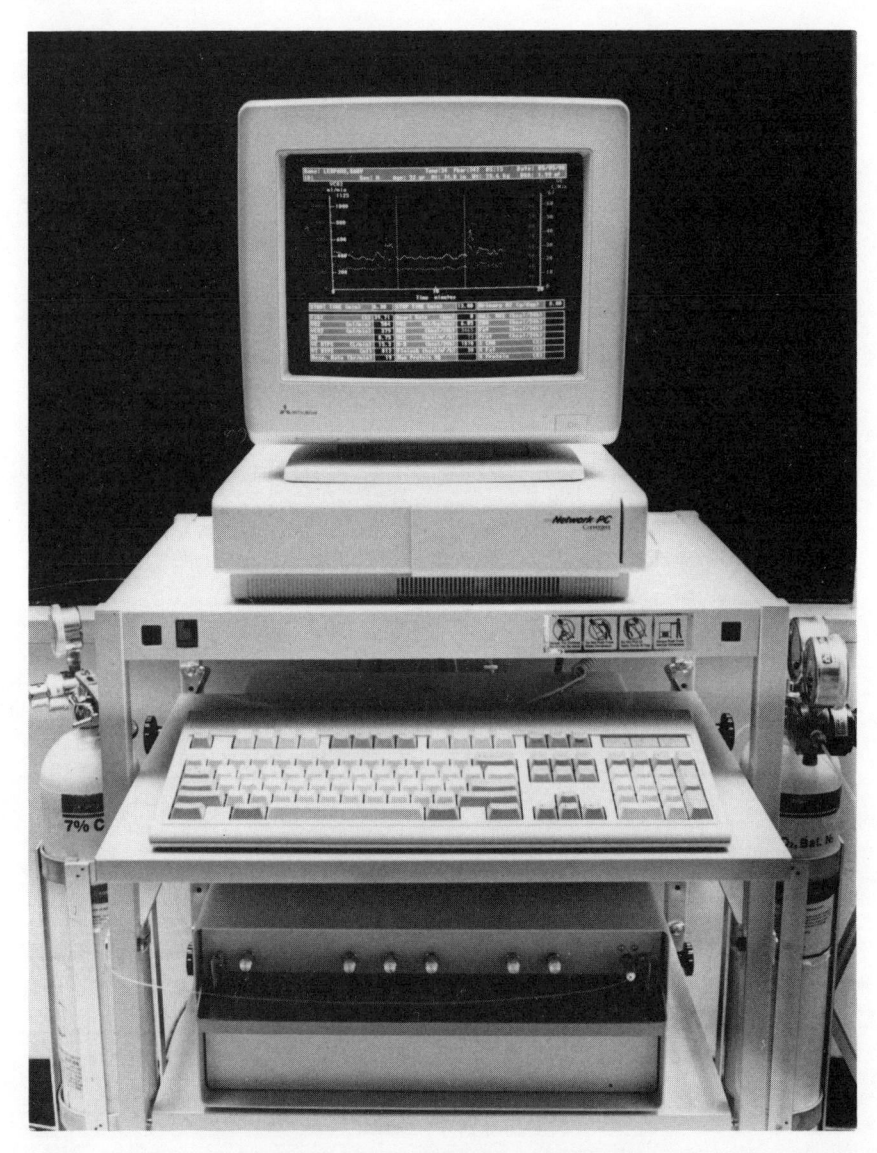

Figure 10. **The Medical Graphics Corporation CCM (Critical Care Monitor).** This metabolic cart provides breath-by-breath measurements for the nutritional assessment of malnourished and/or stressed patients, both on and off ventilators. $\dot{V}O_2$, $\dot{V}CO_2$, FIO_2, and $\dot{V}_E$ are continuously displayed on the screen with each breath, then summarized as mean values per minute at the end of the test run. In addition to these measurements, data output includes RQ, V_T, RR, HR, measured REE (using Weir's formula), and the estimated REE (using the Harris-Benedict formula). When available, the patient's total urinary nitrogen (g/day) can be entered.

SensorMedics Corporation (Figure 11)
1630 South State College Blvd.
Anaheim, CA 92806
Telephone 714/634-0233

Waters Instruments, Inc. (Figure 12)
P.O. Box 6117
2411 7th St. NW
Rochester, MN 55903
Telephone 507/288-7777

Gambro Engstrom (Figure 13)
600 Knightsbridge Parkway
Lincolnshire, IL 60069
Telephone 312/634-6411 or 1-800-558-0555

(4) **Accessory Devices to Collect Expired Air in Spontaneously Breathing Patients.**

  (a) **The mouthpiece, noseclip, and nonrebreathing valve** are useful for short tests, but difficulties may be encountered if measurements are longer than 10 minutes. Some of the problems are failure to obtain a tight seal, collection of saliva in the floor of the mouth, dry throat, jaw fatigue, and inability of the subject to relax.[15] At times the mouthpiece may become so uncomfortable that the patient simply refuses to retain it any longer.

  (b) **The face mask** often presents problems because of the large dead space and the potential for air leaks. A new type of **mouth/face mask** ("VOCA", Hans Rudolph, Kansas City, MO) is ready for marketing and looks most promising from the standpoint of comfort and obtaining accurate measurements (Figure 14, page 55).

  (c) **The head canopy (hood) or "bubble"** is the preferred accessory device, especially for measurements lasting more than 10–15 minutes (Figures 8a, 8b, 15). The head canopy was developed for indirect calorimetry 25 years ago by Kinney and colleagues[91,92] and has many advantages over other methods. The patient's head is enclosed in a rigid, transparent, plastic hood which has a collar to form an airtight seal. Some canopies have large ports on each side so that the patient can scratch, and some have ports for nasogastric tubing and gas monitoring. A pump pulls room air through the canopy at a

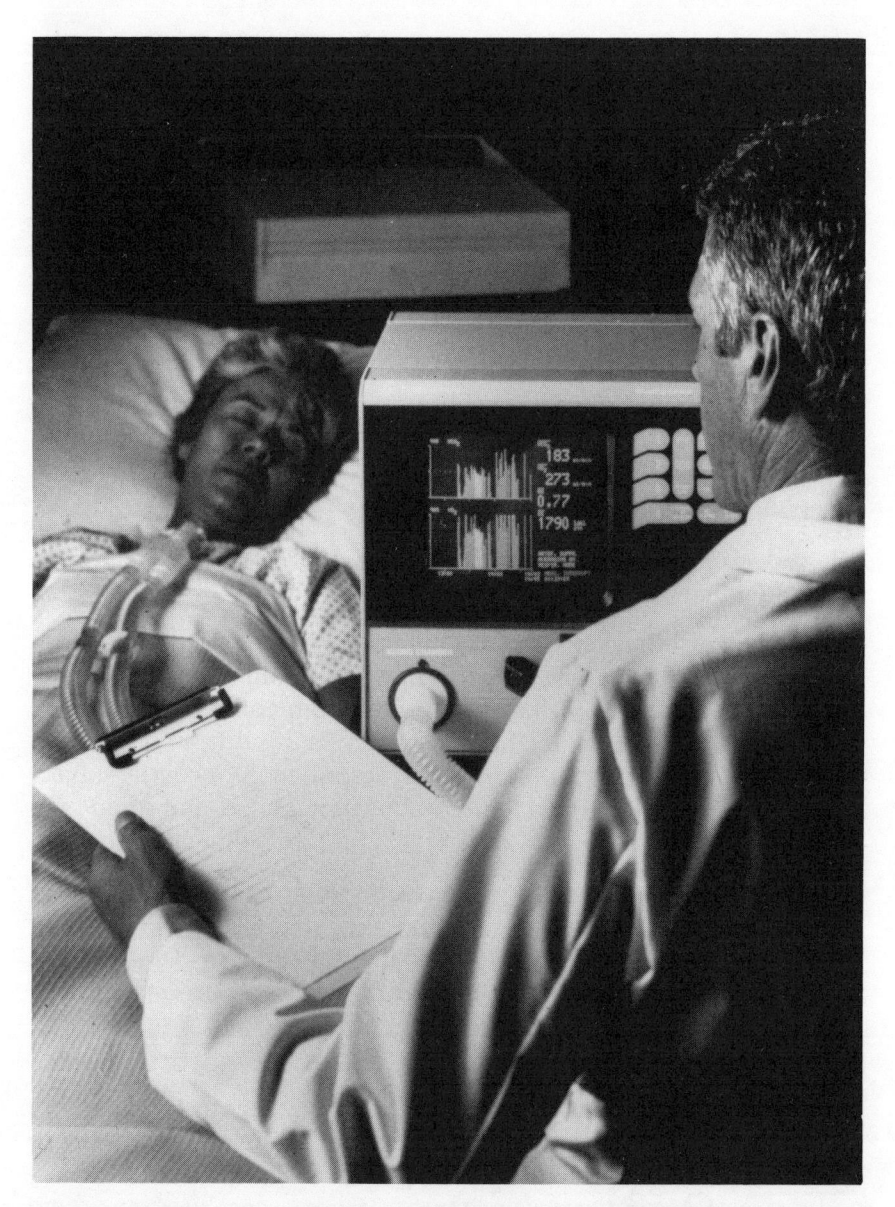

Figure 11. **The SensorMedics Deltatrac Metabolic Monitor.** This compact model measures gas exchange and calculates nutritional needs in both mechanically and spontaneously breathing patients. Data ($\dot{V}O_2$, $\dot{V}CO_2$, and RQ) are continuously monitored and displayed on the screen each minute. The mean values per minute are shown at the end of the test along with the measured REE by indirect calorimetry and the estimated REE by the Harris-Benedict formula.

Evaluating Nutritional Needs

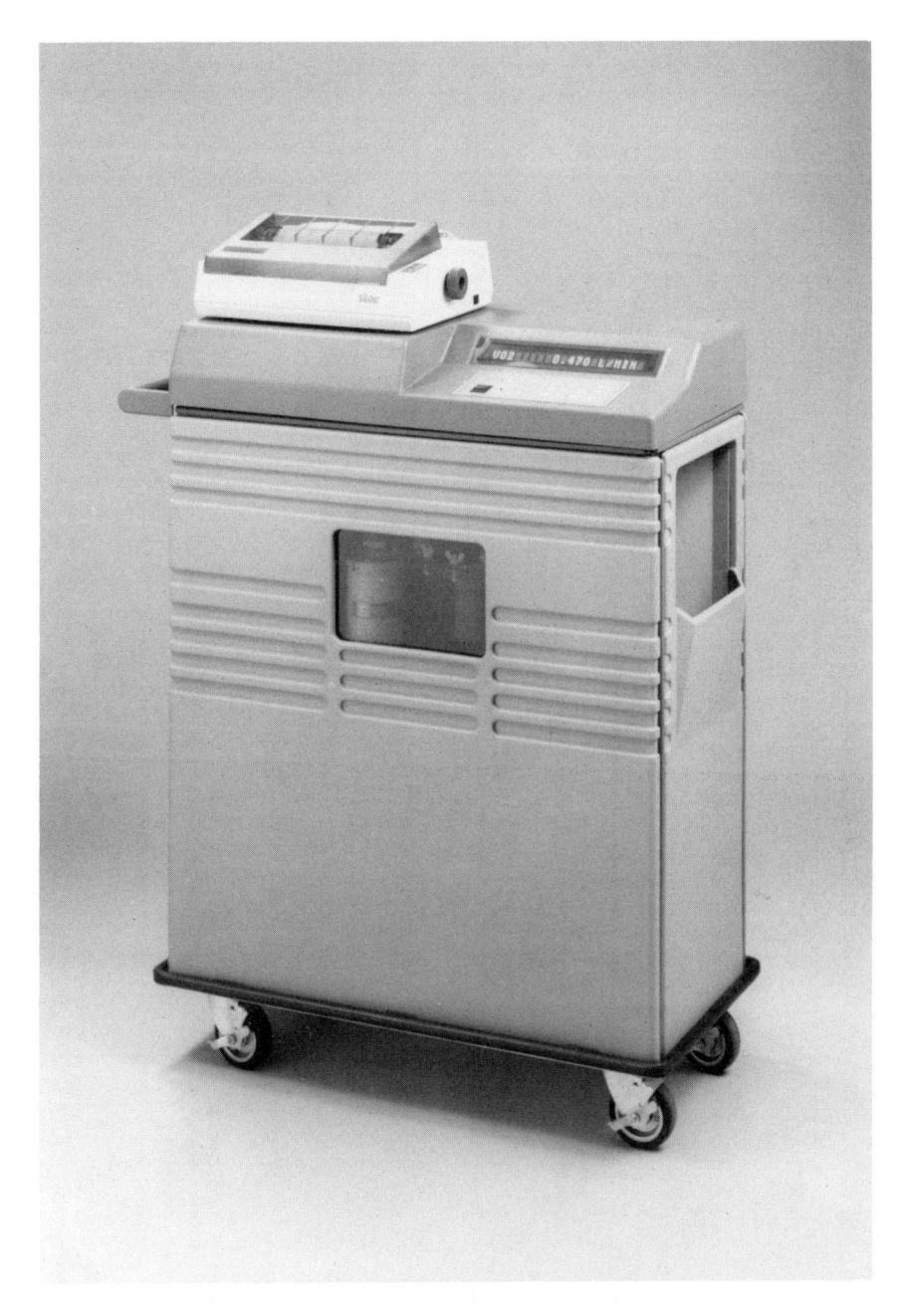

Figure 12. **The Waters MRM-6000 Metabolic Monitoring System.** The instrument is a closed-circuit system that monitors respiratory, metabolic, and indirect calorimetric measurements.

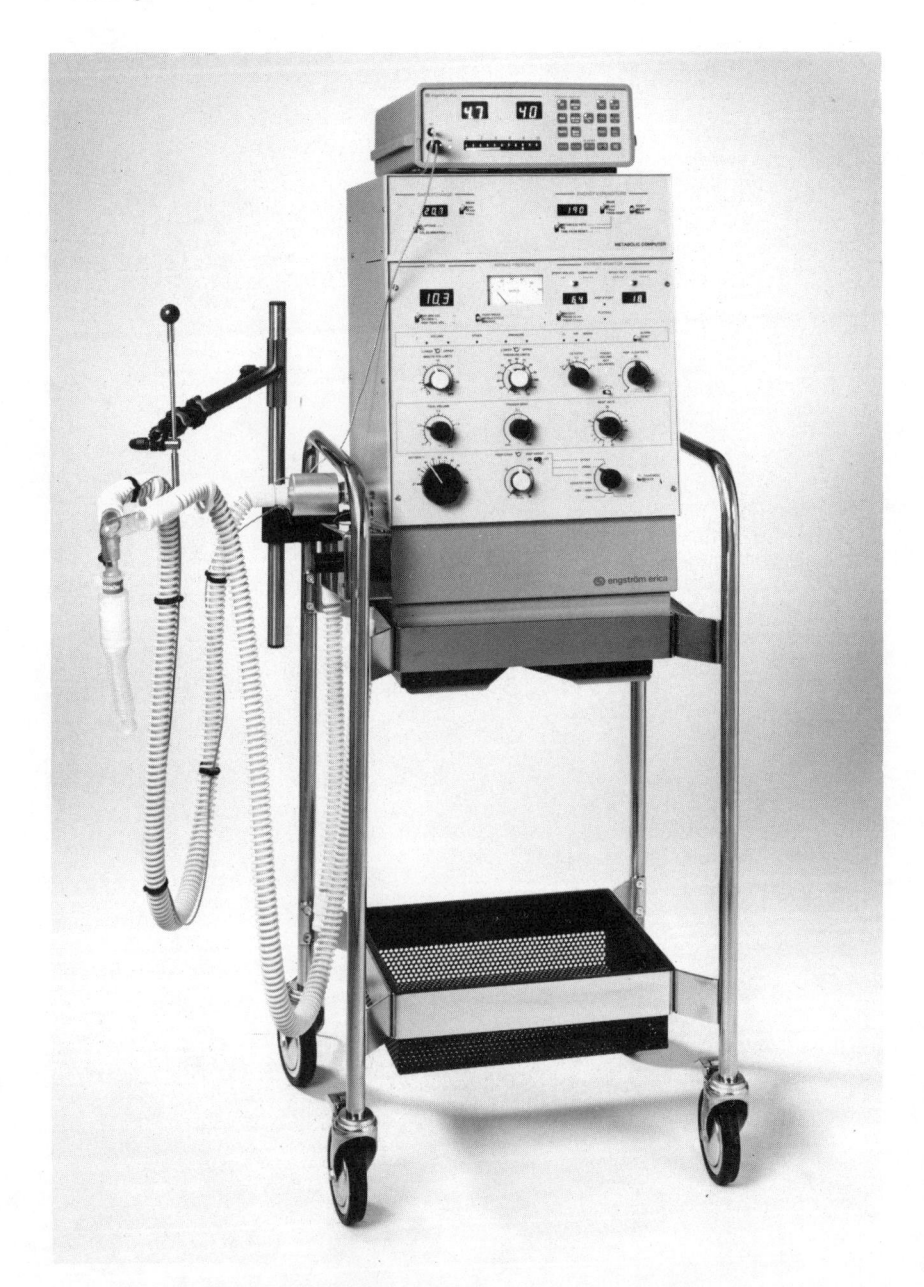

Figure 13. **The Engstrom Erica IV Ventilation/Metabolic System** (Gambrohospal Inc, subsidiary of Gambro Engstrom, Sweden). This combined modular setup is designed to measure oxygen uptake ($\dot{V}O_2$) and carbon dioxide production ($\dot{V}CO_2$) while the patient is being mechanically ventilated, thus eliminating the need for an entirely separate metabolic cart.

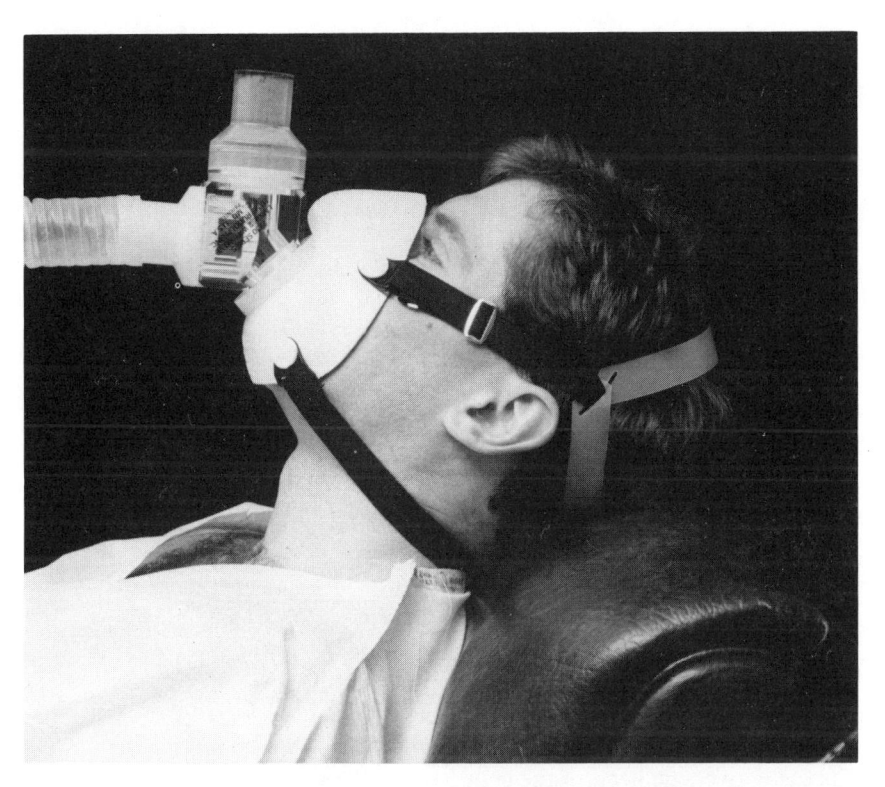

Figure 14. **The Hans Rudolph VOCA mouth/face mask.** This newly designed, comfortable accessory device is ideal for measuring REE in the spontaneously breathing patient. It has the advantage of eliminating jaw fatigue, leakage of air, and pooling of oral secretions. Also the mouth/face mask has a low dead space and is especially applicable for the elderly, the young, and for patients who have loose-fitting dentures. A noseclip is not needed since a partition inside the mask isolates the nose.

continuous flow rate, which is adjusted so that the FCO_2 inside the canopy is kept between 0.0065 and 0.0085. The oxygen uptake ($\dot{V}O_2$) and carbon dioxide production ($\dot{V}CO_2$) are then calculated by computer from the differences in the concentrations of these gases between inspired and expired air, plus the measured air flow through the canopy as opposed to the patient's minute ventilation. Under controlled conditions these measurements are accurate and have none of the inconveniences of other gas collection systems.[93] Recently, Medical Graphics Corporation (St. Paul, MN) introduced an innovative, transparent "bubble" that fits over the subject's head and has several advantages over the older hood or canopy models,

Evaluating Nutritional Needs

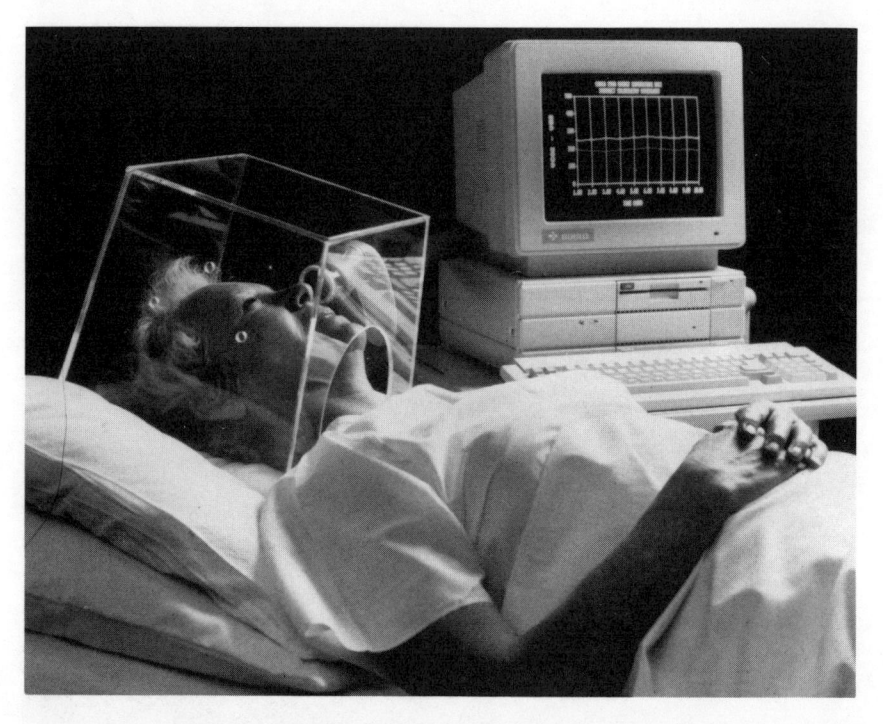

Figure 15. **The SensorMedics Canopy-Blower System.** The lightweight hood fits easily over the head of the spontaneously breathing patient and collects expired air for measurement of gas exchange. Any inconveniences or discomfort from using a mouthpiece is avoided.

including comfort and the capability of carrying out breath-by-breath analysis with great accuracy (Figures 8a, 8b)

(5) **Mechanically Ventilated Patients.** Technical problems are encountered when nutritional assessment by indirect calorimetry is performed in the mechanically ventilated patient. These problems include incomplete mixing of inspired gas, variations in the FIO_2, and the undesirable effects of water vapor, dead space, and pressure fluctuations. To obviate these problems, a **breath-by-breath** system is necessary[94] rather than relying on a mixing chamber where errors as large as ±30% are common.

Close attention must be given to other technical details. For example, the gas sample line must be connected into the patient's breathing circuit as near the ET (endotracheal) tube as possible. The best location is between the "Y" of the ventilator tubing and the ET tube (Figure 16). An airway adapter with a Luer lock

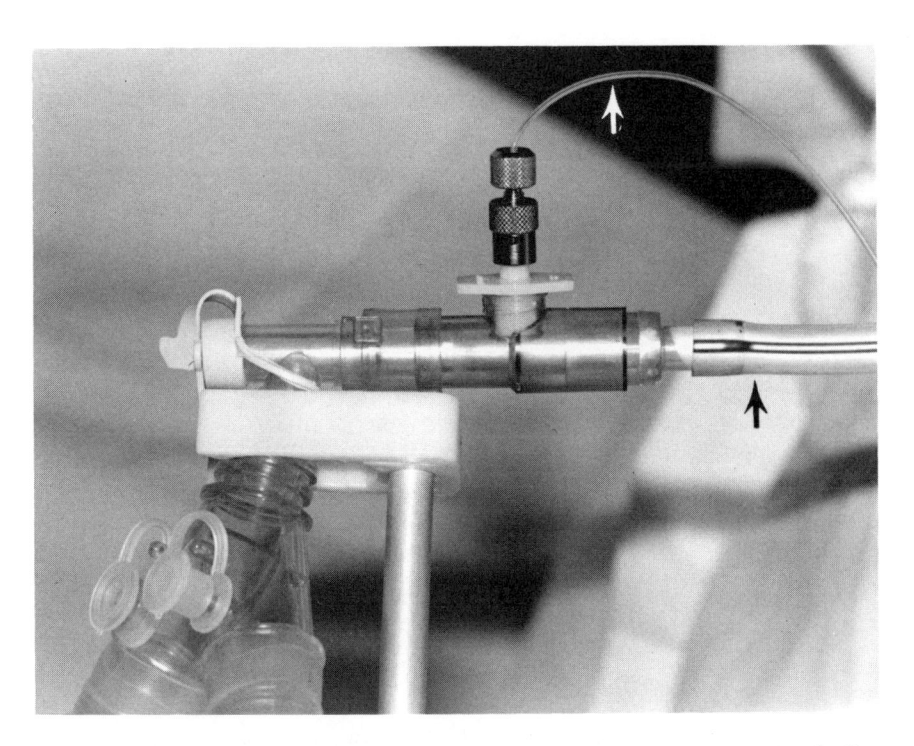

Figure 16. For accurate measurement of gas exchange in the mechanically ventilated patient, the **gas sample line** (light arrow) should be connected adjacent to the endotracheal tube (dark arrow).

connector for the sample line will minimize the dead space. The pneumotachometer (to measure $\dot{V}_E$) is connected downstream from the ventilator on the expiratory line (Figure 17). In *older types* of ventilators, (e.g., MA-1) an isolation valve (Boehringer Part # 8890) is necessary during ventilation to separate the patient's exhaled gas from the continuous flow of the ventilator. *In such instances, positive end-expiratory pressure (PEEP) or continuous positive airway pressure (CPAP) should be turned off during the test.* For patients on any of the *newer models* of ventilators (except the Bear-5), indirect calorimetry can be performed accurately without an isolation valve. The Bear-5 ventilator, however, requires a Boehringer isolation valve because this particular model has a biased flow of 5.0 liters directed to the patient circuit during the expiratory phase. Only by using an isolation valve on the Bear-5 model have we been able to obtain reasonable values for the $\dot{V}O_2$ and $\dot{V}CO_2$; otherwise, the results have been grossly inaccurate.

Evaluating Nutritional Needs

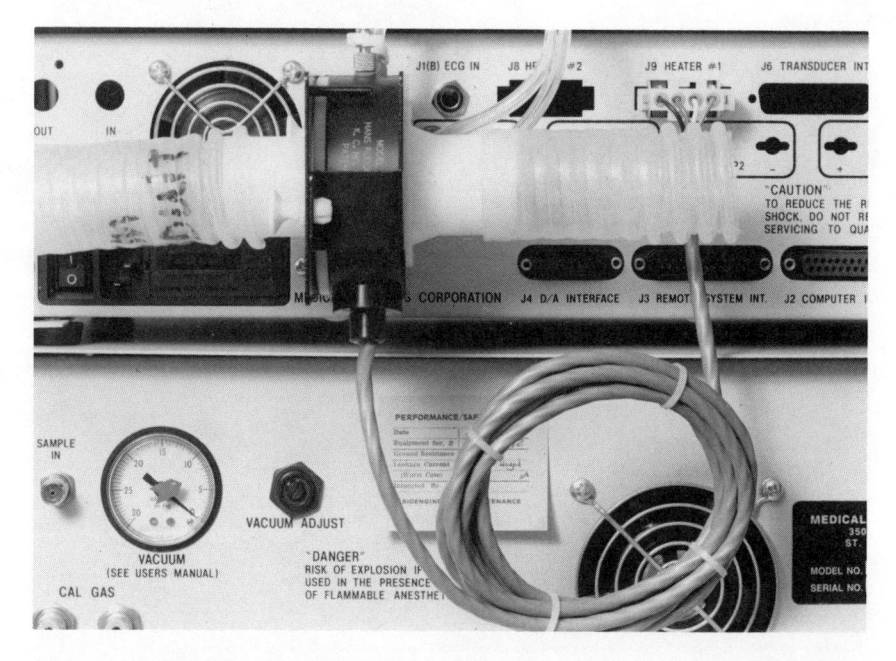

Figure 17. The **pneumotachometer** shown above is located at the rear of Medical Graphics CCM. This device for measuring minute ventilation ($\dot{V}_E$) is connected downstream from the ventilator to the patient's expiratory line.

(6) Sources of error. The following situations may lead to significant errors in indirect calorimetry:

   (a). When FIO_2s are unstable.

   (b). When FIO_2 values are above 0.5–0.6 (see p. 45, item "e").

   (c). When any patient-generated breaths are insufficient in volume to be accepted by the measuring system.[95]

   (d). When air leaks are present in the breathing/ventilator circuit. For patients on ventilators, leaks are more prone to occur at the cuff of the endotracheal tube or the tracheostomy tube, especially if the patient has tracheomalacia.

   (e). When the patient is on hemodialysis. In this situation a sizable amount of CO_2 is removed through the coil.

Evaluating Nutritional Needs

(f). When the patient has had a thoracotomy tube inserted for treatment of a bronchopleural fistula. Significant CO_2 leaks occur via the fistula.[96]

Note: The CO_2 lost (*items e and f*) will alter $\dot{V}CO_2$ and RQ values.

CASE STUDY

PATIENT: G.L., male, 22 years old.

DIAGNOSIS: (1) Acute undifferentiated leukemia with 80% blast cells in the bone marrow.

(2) Opportunistic lung infection (biopsy-culture-proven cephalosporium) that developed immediately following a second course of TADPO (6-thioguanine, Ara-C, daunorubicin, prednisone, and oncovin).

HISTORY: The patient was admitted to the Medical ICU on 4 May 1988, in acute respiratory failure, two weeks after his second course of chemotherapy (TADPO). Vital signs: temperature 39°C, pulse 130/min (sinus tachycardia), respiratory rate 38/min, and blood pressure 164/54 mmHg. Examination of the chest revealed dullness to percussion and decreased breath sounds posteriorly over both lung bases. The heart tones were normal. Chest roentgenograms revealed moderate bilateral lower lobe infiltrates, a 4 cm cavitary lesion in the posterobasal segment of the right lower lobe, and bilateral pleural effusion. On a 50% Ventimask his arterial blood gas values showed a pH of 7.46, PCO_2 27 torr, PO_2 87 torr, and HCO_3 19 mEq. Within 2 hours his respiratory rate rose to 62/min, and the arterial PO_2 decreased to 54 torr. He was intubated and placed on a Servo Ventilator 900 C (Siemens-Elema, Sweden) using assist/control at a respiratory rate of 17/min, a tidal volume of 800 ml, an FIO_2 of 0.40, and zero PEEP. His respirations stabilized at a mean rate of 20/min, and the PO_2 values were in the range of 71–78 torr. Amphotericin B, Imipenem and nutrients were administered via a Hickman line that previously had been placed in the superior vena cava via the right external jugular vein. The patient's respiratory failure seemed to be out of proportion to the moderate degree of lung involvement. Diaphragmatic fatigue was believed to be a factor. His appetite had become increasingly poor over the previous 10 days, and he had lost 4.5 kg in weight. **A nutritional assessment was carried out on 5 May 1988:**

ANTHROPOMETRICS (see Tables 3–11):

Age: 22 years; Sex: male; Height: 188 cm; Wt.: 70 kg; BSA: 1.95 M^2; Usual Wt.: 89 kg

Wrist circumference	17.5 cm (6 7/8″)
Ideal body weight (large frame)	83 kg
Weight as % of ideal body wt.	70/83 × 100 = 84%
Weight as % of usual wt.	70/89 × 100 = 79%
Triceps skinfold (TSF)	5 mm
TSF as a percentile:	10th percentile
Midarm circumference (MAC)	23 cm
Midarm muscle circumference (MAMC)	23 − (3.14 × 0.5) = 21.4 cm
MAMC as a percentile	5th percentile
Interpretation of data	Energy stores—depleted
	Protein stores—depleted

Evaluating Nutritional Needs

LABORATORY TESTS (see Table 12, also pp. 24–34):

White blood cell count	200/mm³ (14th day post TADPO)
Lymphocytes	virtually zero
Serum albumin	2.1 g/dl (low)
Total iron binding capacity (TIBC)	123 mcg/dl (low)
Serum transferrin:	Measured in lab = 91 mg/dl (low) Calculated: (0.68 × 123) + 21 = 105 mg/dl
Creatinine-Height index (CHI)	24 hr. urine creatinine = 1200 mg Normal subject same ht. = 1971 mg 1200/1971 = 61% (low)
Skin tests	Neg. *Candida,* PPD, mumps
Urine urea nitrogen (UUN)	27 g/24 hrs (very high)
Nitrogen balance	$\frac{75}{6.25} - (27 + 4) = -18$g (N loss/24 hrs) = loss of 540–576 g of lean body mass/day (1.0 g N loss = 30–32 g lean body mass)
Other data	phosphorus 3.0 mg/dl, calcium 6.5 mg/dl (ionized calcium normal), potassium 3.9 mg/dl, magnesium 1.6 mg/dl, BUN 27 mg/dl, creatinine 1.5 mg/dl, cholesterol 161 mg/dl, triglycerides 262 mg/dl, hemoglobin 9.7 g/dl, hematocrit 28%

Nutrition

The following data are mean values of the patient's daily intake of energy expressed in kilocalories:

From the 14th to the 8th day prior to mechanical ventilation

	Amount by CVN	Conversion factor	kcal/day	Amount per os	Conversion factor	kcal/day	Total kcal	% of total kcal
CHO	450 g	3.4*	1530	75 g	4.0	300	1830	86%
PRO	75 g	4.0	300	0	4.0	0	300	14%
FAT	0	10.0**	0	0	9.0	0	0	0%

Total = 2130 ± 154

From the 7th to the 4th day prior to mechanical ventilation

	Amount by CVN	Conversion factor	kcal/day	Amount per os	Conversion factor	kcal/day	Total kcal	% of total kcal
CHO	175 g	3.4*	595	200 g	4.0	800	1395	63%
PRO	75 g	4.0	300	0	4.0	0	300	14%
FAT	50 g	10.0**	500	0	9.0	0	500	23%

Total = 2195 ± 112

From the 3rd to the 1st day prior to mechanical ventilation

	Amount by CVN	Conversion factor	kcal/day	Amount per os	Conversion factor	kcal/day	Total kcal	% of total kcal
CHO	350 g	3.4*	1190	0	4.0	0	1190	60%
PRO	75 g	4.0	300	0	4.0	0	300	15%
FAT	50 g	10.0**	500	0	9.0	0	500	25%

Total = 1990 ± 76

*For calculating kcal/day, a conversion factor of 3.4 rather than 4.0 is used for dextrose since it is hydrated (contains a water molecule).
**A conversion factor of 10.0 rather than 9.0 is used for 20% Intralipid since it contains glycerin and an emulsifier (egg yolk

Evaluating Nutritional Needs

On the first day of mechanical ventilation:

Using the Harris-Benedict formula, the patient's resting energy expenditure (REE) was *estimated* to be 1820 kcal/24 hours as shown:

REE = [66.47 + (13.75 × W) + (5 × H)] − [6.76 × A]

   = [66.47 + (13.75 × 70) + (5 × 188)] − [6.76 × 22]

   = 1820 kcal/24 hrs × 1.2 (Activity Factor)

   = 2184 kcal/24 hrs.

On the same day, indirect calorimetry was carried out using a metabolic cart (Critical Care Monitor, Medical Graphics Corp, St. Paul, MN). The following mean data were obtained using three 20-minute, evenly spaced runs throughout the day: $\dot{V}O_2$ = 482 ml/min, $\dot{V}CO_2$ = 358 ml/min, RQ = 0.74. One of the runs is shown in Figure 9, page 49. The patient's REE was *calculated* to be 3274 kcal/24 hrs, using Weir's short formula:

REE = [3.9 ($\dot{V}O_2$) + 1.1 ($\dot{V}CO_2$)] 1.44

   = [(3.9 × 482) + (1.1 × 358)] 1.44

   = 3274 kcal/24 hrs. × 1.1 (Activity Factor)*

   = 3601 kcal/24 hrs (kcal needed)

Comment: Note the large difference between the estimated REE of 1820 kcal/day (adjusted to 2184 kcal/day) and the indirect caloric measurement of 3274 kcal/day (adjusted to 3601 kcal/day). Also observe the low RQ of 0.74, which indicates that exogenous fats are the main oxidative substrate due to lack of caloric intake (starvation) and sepsis. Upon reviewing the data from anthropometry, laboratory tests, and indirect calorimetry, the patient was judged to be hypermetabolic, catabolic, and greatly underfed. Therefore, the energy intake by central venous route was promptly increased from an average of 1990 kcal ± 76 to a mean value of 3510 ± 185 kcal/24 hrs as illustrated on the next page.

*See page 42 and reference 85.

Evaluating Nutritional Needs

Daily energy intake (mean values) from the 1st to the 14th day of mechanical ventilation (assist/control-16, FIO_2 0.35, zero PEEP):

	Amount by CVN	Conversion factor	kcal/day	Amount per os	Conversion factor	kcal/day	Total kcal	% of total kcal
CHO	450 g	3.40	1530	0	4.0	0	1530	43%
PRO	120 g	4.0	480	0	4.0	0	480	14%
FAT	150 g*	10.0	1500	0	9.0	0	1500	43%

*20% lipid emulsion = 2.0 kcal/ml

Total = 3510 ± 185

Twenty-four hours after the above dietary adjustment was made (2nd day of mechanical ventilation), a repeat metabolic evaluation by indirect calorimetry yielded the following data: $\dot{V}O_2$ = 496 ml/min, $\dot{V}CO_2$ = 426 ml/min, RQ = 0.86. Using Weir's short formula, the patient's REE was calculated to be 3460 kcal/day.

Weaning was started on the 11th day of mechanical ventilation and completed on the 14th day. Of interest is the fact that weaning was not successful until the patient's $\dot{V}O_2$ fell below 6.0 ml/kg/min (244 ml O_2/min/m²) while he was being ventilated in the assist/control mode. *More importantly, the % $\Delta \dot{V}O_2$ between mechanical ventilation ($\dot{V}O_2$ assist/control-16) and spontaneous ventilation ($\dot{V}O_2$ wean, SIMV-4) was 12% when expressed as a percent of $\dot{V}O_2$ during mechanical ventilation.* These data agree with the results of Lewis et al[97] who demonstrated that patients with increases in $\dot{V}O_2$ ***less than 15%*** during spontaneous ventilation, compared to $\dot{V}O_2$ during mechanical ventilation, could be weaned within 24 hours of measurement. On 20 May, 1988, the patient was transferred from the ICU to the hematology-oncology unit where he continued to improve.

A repeat laboratory survey on the day of transfer revealed marked improvement compared to the results 2 weeks previously:

LABORATORY TESTS

	5 May 1988 (placed on ventilator)	20 May 1988 (taken off ventilator)
White blood cell count	200/mm^3	13,730/mm^3
Lymphocytes	essent.zero	1,570/mm^3
Serum albumin	2.1 g/dl	2.8 g/dl
Total iron binding capacity	123 mcg/dl	219 mcg/dl
Serum transferrin (lab.)	91 mg/dl	169 mg/dl
Serum transferrin (calc.)	105 mg/dl	170 mg/dl
Creatinine-height index	61%	77%
Skin Tests	negative	positive (4 mm)
Urine urea nitrogen	27 g/24 hrs	12 g/24 hrs
Nitrogen balance	−18 g N/24 hrs	+3.2 g N/24 hrs

Other Data:

Phosphorus	3.0 mg/dl	4.3 mg/dl
Calcium	6.5 mg/dl	8.0 mg/dl
Potassium	3.9 mg/dl	4.3 mg/dl
Magnesium	1.6 mg/dl	2.0 mg/dl
Blood urea nitrogen	27 mg/dl	21 mg/dl
Creatinine	1.5 mg/dl	0.7 mg/dl
Cholesterol	161 mg/dl	176 mg/dl
Triglycerides	262 mg/dl	186 mg/dl
Hemoglobin	9.7 g/dl	10.7 g/dl
Hematocrit	28%	32%

Two days after returning to the hematology-oncology unit, the patient's bowel sounds returned, and supplemental oral feedings were started. TPN was discontinued 5 days later. He gained 4.1 kg over the next 12 days. Continued measurements by indirect calorimetry revealed a decrease in REE (kcal/day). *Appropriate dietary adjustments were made, otherwise excessive caloric intake (overfeeding) could have resulted in unnecessary complications.* Follow-up chest roentgenograms over a 2-week period showed gradual clearing of the pulmonary infiltrates, a decrease in the size of the cavity, and resolution of the pleural effusion. A repeat bone marrow aspiration revealed that he was in remission. Subsequently, the patient's chest roentgenogram completely cleared, and he successfully underwent an allogeneic bone marrow transplant. Currently he is being followed in the hematology-oncology outpatient clinic.

Comment: This case presentation demonstrates the vital role played by nutritional assessment in critical care situations. Poor nutrition, significant protein loss (catabolic metabolism), and underfeeding were felt to be major contributing factors that led to respiratory failure in this 22-year-old man who was undergoing chemotherapy for acute leukemia. Anthropometry, appropriate laboratory tests, and measurement of resting energy expenditure (REE) enabled us to accurately determine the metabolic status of the patient, his total energy needs (kcal/day), and the correct substrate mixture. Thus, with proper nutritional support, he was successfully weaned from mechanical ventilation.

One other important function of indirect calorimetry is the ability to predict whether the patient is ready for weaning from a ventilator. This function is carried out by comparing the patient's $\dot{V}O_2$ during mechanical ventilation with the increased $\dot{V}O_2$ that occurs during weaning (due to the increased work of breathing). Successful weaning usually occurs when the % $\Delta\dot{V}O_2$ between mechanical and spontaneous ventilation is less than 15%, when expressed as a percent of the $\dot{V}O_2$ during mechanical ventilation.[97]

CHAPTER 4
FEEDING THE PATIENT: NUTRITIONAL THERAPY

INTRODUCTION

Before starting nutritional therapy, careful assessment of the patient should be carried out including a medical and dietary history, physical examination, anthropometry, appropriate laboratory tests, and indirect calorimetry (Chapters 2 and 3). After determining the patient's nutritional status, plus caloric and substrate requirements, the next step is to prescribe a ***dietary program*** that will meet the specific needs of each individual. The goal in feeding the critically ill patient is to safely provide enough calories and protein to restore and maintain lean body mass and energy reserves. This chapter briefly reviews the salient features of enteral and parenteral nutrition, delivery methods for feeding (by mouth, tube, or vein), dietary formulations (formulas/infusions), marketing companies, and the composition and purpose of a hospital nutritional support team.

The Standard Routes to Administer Nourishment

(1) Oral

(2) Nasoenteric tube   **Enteral**

(3) Gastrostomy (PEG,PEJ)

(4) Peripheral vein   **Parenteral**

(5) Central vein

Oral feeding is far preferable to any of the other routes, as long as the patient is not prone to aspiration and can digest and absorb major nutrients. To quote Bernard and colleagues: "If the gut works and can be used safely, use it."[19] Yet often the problem is not that patients cannot eat but rather that they cannot willingly eat enough.[53] In such circumstances, intravenous feeding can be successfully combined with oral feeding, making it possible to meet the patient's full nutrient requirements. In catabolic patients with severe protein-calorie malnutrition, enteric feeding by transnasal tube is the preferred method to give nutrients providing there are no contraindications (see below). In fact, enteric feeding by tube is more physiologic than parenteral nutrition and has the following important advantages over the intravenous route: (1) preservation of the gut from disuse atrophy, (2) improved nitrogen balance, (3) faster wound healing, and (4) increased immunocompetence.[19,98-101] Other benefits of enteral nutrition as compared to total parenteral nutrition (TPN) are its safety, convenience, and reduced cost. Unfortunately, situations arise where feeding by the gastrointestinal (GI) tract is not safe, advisable, or possible, in which instances TPN can be lifesaving.

ENTERAL NUTRITION

The advantages, limitations, and techniques for administering enteric feedings are reviewed by Rolandelli and co-workers[101,102] and summarized below. The patient with a functioning GI tract whose oral intake is not completely adequate can be readily managed with oral supplements using liquid formulas. However, if the patient's oral intake does not meet two-thirds of his or her needs, supplemental feedings by nasoenteric tube are indicated.[101]

Nasoenteric Tube Feeding. **For short-term therapy,** insertion of a soft, weighted tip, small-bore tube made of silicone rubber or polyurethane, is the preferred technique.[104] The methodology of tube insertion is discussed in detail by Bernard and co-workers.[19] For maximal protection from aspiration, the tube should be advanced into the duodenum or jejunum. Fluoroscopy is helpful, but at times a gastroscope is needed to position the feeding tube beyond the pylorus. *Long-term enteral nutrition (over 4 weeks)* is best accomplished by percutaneous endoscopic gastrostomy (PEG) or jejunostomy (PEJ) as described below.

INDICATIONS FOR NASOENTERIC TUBE FEEDING[19,101,103]

(1) Neurological disorders (e.g., CVA, demyelinating diseases)

(2) Reduced consciousness or coma

(3) Oropharyngeal or esophageal disorders (e.g., esophageal obstruction)

(4) Inflammatory bowel disease (note: malabsorption may severely limit enteric nutrition)

(5) Hepatic or renal failure

(6) Cardiac cachexia

(7) Respiratory failure (e.g., mechanically ventilated patient with loss of awareness or failure to be weaned)

(8) Multiple organ failure

(9) Trauma, burn, or sepsis

(10) Preoperative preparation or after major surgery (in selected patients)

(11) Neoplasms, radiotherapy, or chemotherapy

(12) Psychological disorders (e.g., anorexia nervosa, depression)

(13) Transition from TPN to TPN + tube feeding, prior to anticipated oral intake

CONTRAINDICATIONS FOR NASOENTERIC TUBE FEEDING[19,101,103]

(1) Intestinal or gastric outlet obstruction (complete or incomplete)

(2) Vomiting or irreversible diarrhea

(3) Gastrointestinal hemorrhage

(4) Severe ileus that cannot be reversed (Patients with mild ileus should be monitored carefully if nasoenteric tube feedings are given.)

(5) Pancreatic or biliary disease (The physician may elect to put the bowel at rest in patients with pancreatic-biliary dysfunction.)

(6) Peritonitis, enterocutaneous fistulae, severe malnutrition

Note: The danger of aspiration is not a contraindication for enteric feeding if the nutrients are delivered into the duodenum or jejunum via tube.

Techniques in Tube Feeding. The delivery of nutrients by tube into the stomach can be performed intermittently or continuously, but placement of the tube into the duodenum or jejunum usually necessitates that the patient *be fed continuously*.[102] By comparison, gastric feeding is often on an intermittent basis, which gives less-ill patients freedom to move about between meals. When continuous tube feeding is administered into the stomach, elevation of the head of the bed 30° to 45° (to help prevent aspiration) sometimes may not be possible in a critically ill patient. When feeding continuously into the small bowel, isotonic solutions (300 mOsm/L) are begun at 25–50 ml/hr, and then the feedings are increased 25 ml/hr every 8 hours until the desired volume is reached.[102] Routinely, hypertonic formulas are diluted to near iso-osmolarity.

Use of a volumetric feeding pump (e.g., Kangaroo-330, Sherwood Medical) reduces the risk of aspiration, is well tolerated, and achieves nutritional goals in a shorter period of time than gravity flow.[100,101] Alarms on these enteric pumps give visual and audible warnings if there is occlusion of the feeding line, if the feeding container is empty, if there is an accidental change in the rate of flow, or if the battery is low. Operational and cleaning instructions are given by the manufacturers. **Note:** To prevent electric shock, one should be sure to unplug the pump before cleaning.

COMPLICATIONS OF TUBE FEEDING[19,98,101-103]

(1) **Diarrhea**—the most common complication; occurs in 10–25% of enterally fed patients[105]

(2) **Nausea and vomiting**—dumping like syndrome; occurs in 10–20% of enterally fed patients[105]

(3) **Aspiration**—the greatest single hazard

(4) **Metabolic imbalances**

   a. hypertonic dehydration due to hyperosmolar nutrients

   b. pseudodiabetes manifested by glycosuria (without acetonuria), osmotic diuresis, and hyperglycemia

(5) **Mechanical problems**

   a. obstruction of the tube

   b. improper placement of the tube

   c. irritation or erosions of the nasopharynx

   d. mucosal erosions of the esophagus or stomach (uncommon)

e. sinusitis

f. esophagitis

PREVENTIVE MEASURES

(1) **Steps to prevent GI symptoms**

   a. Wash hands and keep the equipment clean.

   b. Change the bag and tubing at least once a day; keep prepared bags refrigerated until used.

   c. Dilute the feeding.

   d. Slow the rate of the feeding.

   e. Omit a feeding or two when indicated.

   f. Use antidiarrheal agents as required (Lomotil[R], Imodium[R], Paregoric[R]).

   Note: The patients most likely to have insufficient lactase concentrations in their intestinal mucosa are those with radiation enteritis, inflammatory diseases of the bowel, and resections of the stomach or small bowel.[19]

(2) **Steps to prevent aspiration**

   a. Verify position of the tube *before feedings are started.* One may aspirate for GI contents, but x-ray confirmation is recommended to make absolutely certain that the tube is not in the lung (incidence—0.3%).[106] Lateral curving of the tube on the radiograph indicates placement in the mainstem bronchus. The complications of tube misplacement in the lung are pneumothorax (from tube trauma) and the serious problems that arise from an intrapulmonary feeding. Pneumonia, abscess formation, empyema, hypoxemia, and even death have been reported. The risk for such events is highest in obtunded patients or in those with tracheostomies or endotracheal tubes.

   b. Elevate the head of the bed 30° to 45°.

   c. Feed distal to the pylorus.

   d. In unstable patients with GI symptoms, aspirate the tube before each feeding—a residual of greater than 100 ml is an indication to delay or modify the next feeding. In stable patients, checking for gastric residual once/shift is adequate. Burger and

Adams point out that gastric residuals of 100–150 ml in an asymptomatic patient with normal bowel sounds has little clinical significance.[107]

e. Turn the patient to his or her right side (if possible) to assist gastric emptying.

(3) **Steps to correct metabolic complications**

   a. Treat hypertonic dehydration with fluids, usually by diluting the formula with water.

   b. Treat hyperosmolar, hyperglycemic nonketotic coma with vigorous fluid replacement using hypoosmolar solutions intravenously, usually a 0.45% saline solution plus insulin.

   c. Treat hepatic or renal insufficiency using modified feeding programs and special formulas for enteral (rarely parenteral) nutrition (p. 75).

(4) **Steps to prevent tube problems**

   a. Irrigate the feeding tube with 20 ml of tap water at least three times daily or after each intermittent feeding.

   b. Avoid giving crushed tablets or capsule contents through the tube—*use medications in liquid form whenever possible.*

   c. Flush the tube with 30 ml of water before and after giving each medication.

   d. Give ice chips and topical anesthetics to help prevent tube irritation of the nasopharynx.

   Note: A displaced, malpositioned, or obstructed tube should be replaced without delay.

Gastrostomy. For long-term nutritional support (greater than 5 weeks), a gastrostomy may be carried out. Previously a Stamm gastrostomy was performed, often under general anesthesia.[108,109] The operative time was relatively long, and the increased risk of the procedure was not to be taken lightly.

In 1980, the method of *percutaneous endoscopic gastrostomy (PEG)* was introduced into clinical practice by Gauderer and colleagues.[110] This procedure has greatly facilitated enteral feeding, is comparatively safe (10% complications), and has a low mortality rate of only 1%.[111] For an experienced gastroscopist, the technique is not difficult to learn, can be performed in 30–45 minutes, and does not require a general anesthetic. Using a gastroscope, a *PEG* feeding tube (Ross Laboratories, Columbus, OH) is placed through the stomach and abdominal wall using a *pull* technique. In patients at risk for aspiration (e.g., neurological or oropharyngeal disorders), a jejunostomy tube *(PEJ- or J-tube)* is placed instead. From a technical standpoint, a PEG can be converted to a PEJ. During feedings, the head of the bed should be raised 30° to 45° to prevent aspiration.

The *major complication* of the procedure is infection. Preventive measures consist of using sterile technique, cleaning the patient's mouth with hydrogen peroxide, and stopping H_2-blockers (cemetidine or ranitidine hydrochloride) 24 hours beforehand. Some investigators recommend the prophylactic administration of intravenous cefazolin, 1.0 gram, given one-half hour before the procedure.[112] Other major complications are uncommon and consist of gastric bleeding, hematoma, and aspiration. *Minor complications* (13%) are mainly due to accidentally pulling out the tube, ileus, stomal leak, and tube migration. *Potential contraindications* are a previous subtotal gastrectomy or other surgery in the upper abdomen, pyloric channel obstruction, disease of the anterior gastric wall, situations involving high doses of corticosteroids, and morbid obesity.

Monitoring the Patient/Tidbits. Each critically ill patient on nutritional therapy must be examined daily, weighed, checked for caloric intake, and evaluated for any untoward physical findings or symptoms. One must pay close attention to the patient's metabolic status, protein tolerance, and fluid/electrolyte balance. Monitoring of electrolytes, complete blood counts, nitrogen balance, serum albumin, and so forth, play a vital role in patient management.

In addition to the *prevention of tube feeding problems* already discussed (pp. 71, 72), Bernard,[19] Rolandelli,[102] and co-workers recommend obtaining a daily SMA-6 and a weekly CBC with RBC indices, total iron binding capacity, serum iron, and magnesium. *Other useful tidbits of information are as* follows: (1) In patients being mechanically ventilated, enteral nutrition may protect against stress-induced hemorrhage;[113] (2) In patients who are at risk for aspiration (e.g., those on ventilators), a useful method to detect "silent" aspiration is to add a dye marker (food coloring) to the formula and subsequently check the tracheal aspirates for discoloration; (3) In patients being started on hyperosmolar enteral feedings, especially if the gut has not been used for a while, a common practice is to dilute the formula with water to half strength, then gradually increase to full strength over the next 3–4 days; (4) In patients requiring fluid restriction, the formula strength should be increased before volume is raised; (5) In patients with fat malabsorption, a deficiency often is present in calcium, magnesium and fat soluble vitamins (A, D, E, and K); and (6) In patients who have poor motility of the upper GI tract, gastric emptying may be improved by administering intravenous metoclopramide (Reglan[R]), 10 mg every 6 hours.[102] **Note:** Before giving metoclopramide, it is imperative to make certain that there is no obstruction of the GI tract.

ENTERAL FORMULAS

Two different classifications for enteral formulas are presented here, although neither is entirely satisfactory.

(A) CLASSIFICATION BASED ON COMPOSITION OF THE NUTRIENT (favored by Koruda, Geunter, and Rombeau).[114]

- **(1) Polymeric.** These formulas are complete diets (CHO, PRO, FAT, vitamins, minerals) that can be blenderized whole foods, milk-based, or lactose-free. The lactose-free formulas are reasonably tasteful, comparatively inexpensive, and are the initial choice when GI digestion and absorption are still intact. There is lack of flexibility in these diets because of fixed composition. The liquid formulas usually contain 1 kcal/ml but may be as high as 2–3 kcal/ml. **Examples:** Ensure Plus HN, Osmolite HN, Isocal HCN, Sustacal HC, and Magnacal.

- **(2) Oligomeric.** These formulas are low-residue, complete diets that contain all the essential vitamins and minerals. They consist of *oligo*peptides or amino acids as protein and *oligo*saccharides or disaccharides as carbohydrates, hence the name "oligomeric." The diets are easy to digest, are useful during periods of gut recovery (e.g., GI surgery or ileus), but have the disadvantages of high cost, bad taste, and hyperosmolar composition. Oligomeric formulas are administered by a small-bore nasoenteric tube, however an osmotic diarrhea will develop if the feeding is given too fast. **Examples:** Precision LR, Precision HN, and Vital HN. Special formulas are available for hepatic encephalopathy, renal failure, stress, trauma, and thermal injury (see Special Formulas listed below under *item 4*). **Note:** See p. 80 under item B-1 for a description of elemental formulas.

(3) **Modular.** These diets consist of single or multiple nutrients that may or may not be complete and are used in patients who have special or unusual nutrient requirements. The major disadvantages of these supplemental diets are the high cost, expertise required in their use, and the potential for deficiency states and metabolic complications. **Examples:** *Carbohydrate*: Hycal, ModuCal, Polycose, Sumacal. *Fat*: Microlipid, MCT oil, and Lipomul. *Protein*: Aminess, Casec, ProMed, Pro-Mix, and Propac. *Complete:* Nutri-source (a flexible, modular system of individual nutrient components for tailoring the patient's nutritional support to meet their special needs).

(4) **Special (expensive).**

  (a) **Formulas for hepatic encephalopathy** (Cerra FB, et al: JPEN 9 [3]: 288–295, 1985) contain large amounts of BCAA (branched chain amino acids: leucine, isoleucine, valine) and low amounts of methionine and aromatic amino acids (tryptophan, tyrosine, phenylalanine). Use of these formulas does not appear to improve survival. **Examples:** Hepatic-Aid and Travasorb Hepatic. HeptAmine is for parenteral use. **Note:** In alcoholism with acute hepatic decompensation, therapy also mandates giving supplemental multivitamins (p. 98), essential trace metals, appropriate minerals (pp. 99–101), electrolytes as needed (pp. 32, 33, 89–91, 97, 98), and the careful administration of fluids (pp. 88, 121). The cautious use of medium- and short-chain triglycerides may have some beneficial effect. Generally, patients with hepatic dysfunction should not receive more than 40–50 g PRO/day. Furthermore, amino acid administration should be stopped if the patient becomes stuperous.

  (b) **Formulas for acute renal failure** (e.g., acute tubular necrosis) are used chiefly during the pre-dialysis period, hoping to avoid hemodialysis. Theoretically, their purpose is to decrease urea production by recycling nitrogen into the synthesis of nonessential amino acids. These formulas contain essential amino acids (as the source of nitrogen) plus histidine, ample CHO calories, some fat, and scant or no electrolytes. They are lactose-free, hyperosmolar, and not very palatable. **Examples:** Amin-Aid and

Travasorb Renal (usually given by feeding tube). RenAmin and NephrAmine are for parenteral use. **Note:** Special formulas (e.g., Magnacal or Resource Plus) are employed when renal failure is chronic and dialysis is ongoing. Other dietary and intake modifications in chronic renal failure include restriction of protein and phosphate; controlled intake of Na, K, Mg, and free water; also the administration of supplemental vitamin D, calcium salts and phosphate-binding preparations.

(c) **Formulas for stress, trauma, and burns** are high in BCAA. The amino acids used in these hypermetabolic states act as a substrate for both anabolism and energy. The nonprotein calories are provided as CHO (maltodextrins) and as FAT (MCT and soy oil) at a calorie to nitrogen ratio between 80:1 and 100:1. These formulas are hyperosmolar (675–910 mOsm/kg H_2O) and have a caloric density of 1–1.2 kcal/ml.
Examples: Traum-Aid HBC, Stresstein, Criticare HN and Isotein HN.

Several comments are indicated regarding the enteral feeding of burn patients. First, and most important, feeding should be started as soon as the gut is working! A notable feature of *early feeding* (usually by nasoenteric tube) is the prevention of gastrointestinal bleeding and more rapid reversal of the hypermetabolic state. During the acute phase, Curreri and colleagues[73] recommend a protein intake of approximately 2–4 g/kg/day plus adequate multivitamins, including 1–2 g/day of vitamin C. In a burn of moderate to severe degree, low serum albumin levels cannot be corrected to normal (regardless of protein intake) until the denuded skin area is covered. The use of a *high fiber formula such as Jevity* has helped our patients to maintain normal bowel function. Jevity also has a high level of quality protein (total calorie/nitrogen ratio = 150:1), is lactose and gluten free, has MCTs as 50% of the fat system, and is fortified with vitamins, minerals, and trace elements. Our standard procedure is to combine Jevity and Osmolite HN in a 1:1 mixture which has the advantage of high nitrogen and fiber content at a reduced cost. The patients are weighed daily and careful attention paid to their fluid balance. An attempt is made to maintain the patient's weight within 10% of his or her pre-burn weight.

(d) **Formulas for respiratory failure** have a high FAT to CHO ratio in order to reduce CO_2 production and lessen ventilatory requirements. **Note:** In nutritional repletion of COPD patients, it is advisable to *slowly increase caloric intake* while carefully monitoring the respiratory rate, arterial blood gases, body weight, and (if ambulatory) the response to exercise. In addition to the harmful effects of a high CHO load, patients with marginal respiratory function should not receive excessive amino acids (PRO) because of the resulting increase in ventilatory drive with a rise in $\dot{V}O_2$ and $\dot{V}_E$. The reader is referred to a broad review on nutritional support and respiratory function by Askanazi (editor) in Clin Chest Med 7: 1–152, 1986.

(e) **Formula for insulin and noninsulin dependent diabetes** (recently introduced) has a high-fiber, high FAT to CHO ratio, designed to improve blood glucose in patients with TYPE I and TYPE II diabetes. Lower plasma triglyceride values and lower very-low-density lipid levels have been reported[115,116] (Garg A, et al: N Engl J Med 319: 829–834, 1988; also Davidson MB, et al: Clinical Research 37: 140A, 1989.) **Example:** Glucerna (50% FAT, 33.3% CHO, 16.7% PRO). Of the CHO calories, 22% are glucose polymers, 7.1% fructose, and 4.2% soy fiber. The formula has a calorie/nitrogen ratio of 150:1, a low osmolality of 375 mOsm/kg water, and a caloric density of 1.0 Cal/ml. **Note:** One of the beneficial effects of fiber is to alleviate diarrhea and constipation.

(f) **Formulas for acute and chronic pancreatitis** vary according to the condition of the patient.[19] Initially, patients with *acute pancreatitis* (or biliary dysfunction) require IV fluids, nasogastric suction, and meperidine. Infusions may be given by peripheral vein consisting of synthetic crystalline amino acids, electrolytes, dextrose, and fat emulsions. Generally TPN is *not* required unless the acute process is slow to resolve and prolonged bowel rest becomes necessary. During recovery, the patients are started on oral feedings in gradually increasing amounts. The diet is high in CHO, high in PRO, and restricted in FAT to no more than

60 g/day. Nonprotein calorie sources consist of medium-chain triglycerides (MCT) and glucose oligosaccharides (glucose polymers 2–10 molecules long).

Most patients with **chronic pancreatitis** are alcoholics. In such situations, oral diets may be tried at the discretion of the physician, but one should keep in mind that the only way to completely put the pancreas at rest is to utilize TPN. *A reasonable oral nutritional program is to give frequent, small feedings that are low in fat (use MCT), to avoid stimulants (coffee, tea), and to administer a pancreatic enzyme supplement (pancrelipase) such as Cotazym (Organon), Pancrease (McNeil), or Viokase (Robbins).* At times it may be necessary to place a nasoenteric tube in the small bowel of patients who will not voluntarily take in enough nutrients by mouth to meet their tremendously increased metabolic needs. The tube formulas are low in FAT, high in CHO, and contain free amino acids or peptides.

TPN is indicated in patients with persistent pancreatitis (over 5 days), hemorrhagic pancreatitis, or those with postoperative pancreatic pseudocysts, fistulas, or abscesses. Bernard et al[19] recommended TPN therapy that supplies PRO 1.5 g/kg/day, with the nonprotein energy source made up of 70% CHO and 30% FAT. *There appears to be no danger of stimulating the pancreas by giving IV lipid emulsion since the chylomicrons are metabolized peripherally by tissue lipases.*[117]

(g) **Formulas for cardiac cachexia** usually are modular or fixed in composition, low in sodium, and contain 1–2 kcal/ml. The following therapeutic modes have been reviewed by Quinn and Askanazi (*Crit Care Clinics* 3 [1]: 167–184, 1987):

   i. Depending upon gut absorption and patient tolerance, 6 small oral feedings may be given daily.

   ii. For patients with severe anorexia, continuous tube feedings may be employed.

   iii. Parenteral nutrition is used if malabsorption is a problem.

   iv. More concentrated formulas may be used for patients requiring fluid restriction, but feeding adjustments may be necessary if diarrhea occurs.

v. Often increased amounts of protein are required because of malabsorption and/or excessive urinary loss, however, the goal of achieving zero or positive nitrogen balance may have to be modified if the cardiac patient also has renal insufficiency.

vi. MCTs may be substituted for LCTs for patients with fat malabsorption.

vii. More complex starches may be utilized for patients with glucose intolerance.

viii. Vitamin and mineral deficiencies should be corrected promptly.

ix. Diuretics are given plus cardiac medications to handle preload and afterload.

x. Sodium intake is restricted to less than 2 g/day, and fluids are restricted to 1–1.5 L/day.

Note: Preoperative alimentation (2 weeks) can improve the operative outcome for malnourished cardiac patients who are scheduled to have major surgery. For the survival of cardiac transplant patients, adequate nutrition is absolutely essential. Thus, a concerted effort should be made to restore the patient to an anabolic state prior to surgery. Peripheral alimentation, nasoenteric tube feedings or even (in some instances) placement of central lines for TPN may be necessary. Energy needs usually are 1.5 time the basal energy requirement (Hastillo A, Hess ML: *J Crit Illness* 4 [10]: 34–44, 1989).

(B) CLASSIFICATION BASED ON COMPLETE VS INCOMPLETE DIETS[19,36]

(1) Complete diets furnish the recommended dietary allowances for normal and many undernourished people. The required nutrients may be categorized as follows: (a) *Blenderized* (Compleat and Vitaneed), (b) *Milk-based* (Meritene and Sustagen), (c) *Lactose-free* (Isocal, Osmolite, Enrich, Ensure, and Sustacal), (d) *Hydrolyzed protein* (Criticare HN, Vital

HN, and Travasorb), (e) *Crystalline amino acids* plus glucose oligosaccharides and safflower oil (Vivonex T.E.N.), (f) *Specialized formulations* (Traumacal, Pulmocare, and Glucerna). **Note:** *Elemental formulas* contain amino acids (or protein hydrolysates), MCTs, and simple sugars. Usually they are given by nasogastric tube. Absorption takes place in the upper intestine, making the formulas ideal for patients with malfunction of the GI tract, Crohn's disease, short bowel syndrome, and intestinal or rectal fistulas. **Examples:** Osmolite HN, Travasorb HN, Vital HN, Isotein HN.

(2) **Incomplete diets** are formulated to replace dietary deficiencies that may occur with specific diseases or injury, e.g., renal or hepatic failure and trauma. These diets contain specialized amino acids (high in branched-chain and essential amino acids), glucose oligosaccharides, maltodextrins, sucrose, and sunflower, soy, or MCT oils. Their osmolarity is from 590 to 900 mLsm, and they contain 1.1 to 2.0 kcal/ml. **Examples:** Travasorb Renal, Travasorb Hepatic, Amin-Aid, Hepatic-Aid, and Traum-Aid.

PARENTERAL NUTRITION
HISTORICAL BACKGROUND

The fascinating drama of parenteral nutrition unfolds one act at a time, slowly (and painfully) at the beginning, then rapidly advancing for the past 20 years. The final scene is yet to come. In his excellent article on amino acids, Stegink[118] reviewed the history of parenteral nutrition, which is as follows:

1656– Sir Christopher Wren[119] injected nutrients (ale, wine) and drugs (opium) into the veins of dogs using a goose quill attached to a pig's bladder.

1882– Latta[120] administered saline infusions into the veins of patients with cholera.

1886– Biedl and Kraus[121] were the first to give dextrose solutions intravenously to humans.

1904– Abderhalden and Rona[122] were among the first to inject a solution of enzymatically digested protein, consisting of peptides and amino acids.

1913– Henriques and Andersen[123] infused a solution of hydrolyzed

Feeding the Patient

goat muscle protein (plus salt and glucose) by continuous IV drip into goats for 16 days, maintaining their normal weight.

1935– Holt and colleagues[124] were probably the first to use lipid emulsions.

1937– Elman[125] reported substantial regeneration of plasma proteins in dogs after infusions of an amino acid preparation (hydrolysate of casein, tryptophan, and cystine plus 5% glucose solution). This beneficial result did not occur when the animals were given only 10% glucose.

1939– Elman and Weiner[126] reported the first infusion of protein hydrolysate solutions into adult humans, and Shohl et al[127] reported similar studies in infants using an enzymatic hydrolysate of casein.

1940s– The only common intravenous infusion for nutrition during this period was 5% dextrose and water, often given in amounts of 2–3 liters daily.[128]

1940– Schoenheimer and Rittenberg[129] demonstrated the dynamic nature of body nitrogen metabolism, namely that body proteins were in a state of flux, being continually synthesized and degraded.

1944– Helfrick and Abelson[130] reported the first successful total parenteral feeding of a 5-month-old infant with marasmus using IV infusions of 5% glucose, 10% casein hydrolysate, and a crude lipid emulsion.

1965– Mueller[131] stated that there was **no safe IV fat emulsion** available in the United States! Toxic reactions to lipid emulsions date back to their early clinical trials in the 1950s. In 1965, Lipomul*, which consisted of cottonseed oil with soybean lecithin and polymers, was removed from the market because of serious adverse effects. The untoward reactions (overloading syndrome) consisted of fever, abdominal pain, anorexia, anaphylactic reactions, coagulation defects, thrombocytopenia, depressed hematopoiesis, liver dysfunction with hepatosplenomegaly, and persistent hyperlipidemia.[132,133]

1967– **A giant step for mankind!** Dudrick and his co-workers[134] were successful in maintaining the normal growth and de-

*Upjohn Co., Kalamazoo, MI

velopment of beagle puppies who, as the sole source of their nutrition, were infused for up to 36 weeks with hypertonic glucose-protein hydrolysate solutions into the superior vena cava. Thus entered the age of **total parenteral nutrition (TPN)**. *The results of this study were so dramatic that the IV hyperalimentation technique using a central vein was immediately adapted for human use.*[135-137]
Since then there have been continued improvements in the composition of the parenteral solutions,[118] especially in the amino acid and lipid content. **Note:** The reader may wish to review the fascinating story of Dudrick's original work, as told by himself 10 years later[138] (Dudrick SJ: The genesis of intravenous hyperalimentation. *JPEN* 1 (1): 23–29, 1977).

1975– **Eureka!** The first successful fat emulsion, named *Intralipid*‡ (Cutter Laboratories, Inc., Berkeley, CA), was approved for human parenteral use in the United States and consisted of soybean oil and egg yolk phospholipid emulsions. Four years later *Liposyn* (Abbott Laboratories, N. Chicago, IL) was introduced and consisted of an emulsion of safflower oil and egg yolk phospholipids.

INTRAVENOUS NUTRITION (PERIPHERAL/CENTRAL)

PERIPHERAL VENOUS NUTRITION

For short term therapy, nutrition can be provided via a peripheral vein when the patient cannot eat by mouth or cannot eat enough to meet energy requirements. Also, peripheral venous nutrition (PVN) may be considered when enteric tube feeding has failed or is contraindicated (see "Contraindications for Tube Feeding" on page 69).[139] *Still, one must not lose sight of the fact that large amounts of energy to meet greatly increased nutritional needs cannot be supplied solely by the peripheral venous system because of osmolarity restrictions and water-tolerance limitations.*

The quintessential candidate for PVN (of expected short duration) is the patient with inadequate oral intake whose diet can be augmented by the peripheral venous route until full enteral support is achieved. PVN, as the only source of energy, routinely can be carried

‡A product of Kabivitrum, Inc., which currently is being distributed by Clintec Nutrition Co., Deerfield, IL. Of historical interest—this product was used previously in Europe for years.

out for 4–7 days in patients who are small in stature, have good veins for easy access, and have relatively low REEs (resting energy expenditures). Only on **rare** occasions has PVN been given at our medical center for as long as 10–12 days.

The name of the game is preservation of the peripheral vein. As a rule of thumb, PVN solutions provide 100 mOsm/L for each percent of amino acids without electrolytes (125 mOsm/L with electrolytes) and 50 mOsm/L for each percent of dextrose. *Thus, to calculate the osmolarity of an amino acid + dextrose mixture*: 500 ml of 8.5% amino acids added to 500 ml of 20% dextrose = a final concentration of 4.25% amino acids + 10% dextrose = $(4.25 \times 100) + (10 \times 50)$ = 925 mOsm/L. Intravenous fat emulsions provide 260–350 mOsm/L for both 10% and 20% preparations. Blood has an osmolarity of 300 mOsm/L which theoretically means that solutions of 250–500 mOsm/L can be given intravenously without any problems. Actually, in clinical practice these levels can be exceeded. Single vein longevity of 3–7 days has been demonstrated using *final infusates* of 900–980 mOsm/L, but it is not prudent to go beyond these levels.[140] One more important tidbit—in addition to supplying calories and essential fatty acids, *the continuous, simultaneous infusion of fat emulsion in patients on TPN (PRO + CHO) has another paramount advantage, namely a significant reduction in thrombophlebitis*. This beneficial effect (extended use of the vein) is due to dilution of the *hypertonic* amino acid + dextrose solution by the *isotonic* lipid emulsion.

Assuming the patient's peripheral veins are in good condition, PVN is accomplished by inserting a small, plastic catheter into a newly selected vein. The IV catheter is attached to extension tubing that has a *Y connector* at the proximal end for administration of the amino acid + dextrose solution at one port and fat emulsion at the other port. The lipid port has a single *one-way valve* that prevents reflux contamination of the emulsion. Otherwise, the lipid bottle and line should be positioned higher than the amino acid-dextrose container so that the fat emulsion (lower specific gravity) will not be taken up into the amino acid-dextrose line.

CENTRAL VENOUS NUTRITION/TPN
INDICATIONS

By rule of thumb, total parenteral nutrition (TPN) via the superior vena cava is the route of choice when energy requirements are more than **2400 Calories** per day for a period of more than 6–7 days.[141] In this manner, higher concentrations of nutrient can be given to achieve total nutritional support. There are a number of indications for TPN, the most important being the combination of *malnutrition* with significant loss of fat and moderate to severe *stress*. Early TPN (within only a few days) should be initiated for patients under stress who have malfunction of the GI tract and for whom the risk continues for further malnutrition.[142]

THE SEVERE STRESSES ARE AS FOLLOWS:

(1) Sepsis, early and late

(2) Multiple trauma

(3) Head injury

(4) Extensive burns (over 50% of the body surface area).

> **Note:** Albumin levels less than 2.5 g/dl are associated with severe stress.

THE MODERATE STRESSES ARE AS FOLLOWS:

(1) Infection

(2) Significant hemorrhage

(3) Major surgery

(4) Unrelenting pancreatitis

(5) Inflammatory bowel disease

JENSEN AND BISTRIAN[142] GIVE THE FOLLOWING INDICATIONS FOR TPN:

(1) Severe malnutrition

(2) Severe stress (see the four major items above)

(3) Any combination of moderate malnutrition + stress

(4) Loss of GI tract function (likely to continue more than 5–7 days) + stress

(5) Malabsorption of the GI tract (e.g., radiation enteritis, massive small-bowel resection, inflammatory bowel disease, mesenteric thrombosis, enterocutaneous fistulas, small-bowel obstruction due to adhesions)

(6) Bone marrow transplantation

(7) Preparation for cancer surgery or for other types of major surgery (in the presence of significant hypoalbuminemia + moderate stress)

(8) Acute pancreatitis, slow to resolve

Note: Also included in the list are disastrous postoperative complications, acute renal failure (acute tubular necrosis), hepatic insufficiency (selected cases), and coma.[19,139]

TECHNIQUES FOR ADMINISTERING TPN

General Comments. For total parenteral nutrition (TPN), single lumen and multichannel central venous catheters are available. Without a doubt, catheters with a *single* channel are preferred since the danger of infection is reduced. However, recent literature suggests that meticulous technique will provide a low rate of infection for both single and multiple lumen catheters.[143] We do *not* use multichannel catheters except in exceptional situations (e.g., bone marrow transplantation) where it is convenient to use two or three channels to inject chemotherapeutic agents and antibiotics separately from the feeding channel. *Because of the great danger of infection, another helpful dictum is to* **never** *draw a blood sample from a central venous catheter unless absolutely necessary.* But on *rare* occasions, when the need is urgent and definitely no other alternative is available, the physician-in-charge may order the TPN stopped momentarily and a sample obtained for analysis.

Cannulation of the Central Vein. The standard access routes to the superior vena cava are the ***internal jugular vein*** (supraclavicular approach) and the ***subclavian vein*** (infraclavicular approach). Catheterization of the subclavian vein is the usual route at our medical center, although sometimes we utilize the internal jugular vein. This latter approach virtually eliminates the risk of pneumothorax; however, the patient may be more prone to infection since one cannot make an occlusive seal at the site of catheter insertion. Also, the internal jugular route may not be possible because of previous surgery in the area, local infection, neck injury, thrombosis, or difficult entry to the vein. To cannulate the internal jugular or subclavian vein, the patient is placed in Trendelenburg position with a 10° to 15° head down tilt to prevent air embolism. In this position one may observe if there is good filling of the external jugular veins, which helps to determine the patient's state of hydration. A chest x-ray is taken to make certain that the tip of the catheter is in the superior vena cava. For those who want to review the technical aspects of central vein cannulation in detail, I enthusiastically recommend articles by Jensen and Bistrian,[144] Bone,[145] Vander Salm,[146] and Freis.[147]

Catheter Care. Every effort must be made to eliminate infection. Dressings and IV tubing should be changed daily if indicated—a wet dressing must be changed promptly. Routinely we change dressings at least three times a week. A mask and gloves are worn. Povidone-iodine ointment is applied at the insertion site, and an *occlusive dressing* is applied whenever possible. As an additional protection against bacterial contamination, an in-line filter may be used for the amino acid + dextrose infusion, while FAT is piggybacked *distal* to the filter.

Catheter Complications. An indwelling catheter in a central vein acts as a foreign invader. Thus, the physician must be constantly on the alert for catheter related sepsis. One of the first signs of infection may be *glucose intolerance.* Other signs or symptoms of sepsis include chills, fever, drop in blood pressure, mental changes, and leukocytosis with a shift to the left. *When infection is suspected, our routine is to take cultures for aerobes and anaerobes from the following sites:* (1) through the line, (2) from the catheter tip, (3) from the peripheral blood, and (4) from any drainage at the place of insertion. If infection develops, the physician has the option either to reinsert a new catheter at the same site by sliding it over a preinserted guidewire or else to cannulate the vena cava from a new site on the opposite side (via subclavian or internal jugular vein). If the old catheter is culture-positive at its tip, then one has no choice but to use another access site. Catheter sepsis accompanied by positive blood cultures (frequently *Staphylococcus aureus, S. albus,* or *Candida albicans*) is a serious complication of TPN that demands immediate attention! Also if blood cultures remain positive after the catheter is withdrawn, then antibiotic therapy is required for at least 7–14 more days.

Other technical complications encountered in placing a central venous catheter for TPN (especially via the subclavian vein) are as follows: pneumothorax (occurs in up to 5% of the procedures), puncture or laceration of the subclavian artery, hematoma, hemothorax, hydrothorax (when the formula is accidentally administered into the pleural cavity), chylothorax (from laceration of the thoracic duct by a left side approach), nerve injury (phrenic, vagus, brachial plexus) and several rare complications that include air or catheter embolism, septic thrombosis, and cardiac tamponade.[19,145-148] The reader is referred to an excellent paper by Jensen and Bistrian on preventing and managing complications of TPN.[149]

Extended TPN. If long-term TPN is anticipated (e.g., TPN at home), good results are uniformly achieved using a *silastic Hickman catheter.* Besides TPN, other uses of a Hickman catheter are for prolonged intravenous chemotherapy and/or antibiotic therapy. Operating in a sterile field, our routine is to insert the catheter into the superior vena cava via the external jugular vein* and subcutaneously tunnel it downward 6–10 cm from the cannulation site to exit on the anterior chest wall medial to the nipple (Figure 18). A small Dacron cuff, located near the skin exit of the catheter, is effective in preventing the spread of infection. Hickman catheters are easy to manage, more comfortable for the patient, and are far less likely to result in complications such as thrombosis and sepsis. *Broviac* and *Groshong* catheters are also available for long-term nutritional support.

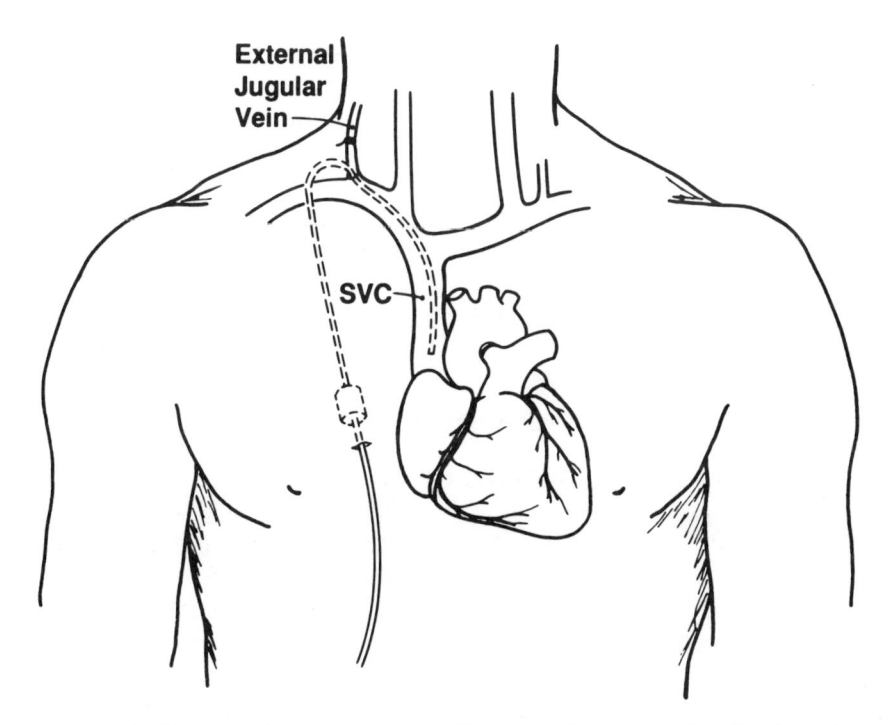

Figure 18. The artist's drawing above illustrates **insertion of a silastic catheter for prolonged TPN.** Modified from Al-Jurf AS, Younoszai H,[166] with permission.

*Alternate routes to the SVC are the internal jugular vein, cephalic vein, or the subclavian vein (listed in the order of preference).

In spite of the excellent record of Hickman catheters in extended TPN, one must always be on guard for complications. *If infection occurs, the standard of care at the University of Iowa Hospitals and Clinics is to attempt sterilization with antibiotics before removing the catheter.* Any one of the following drug combinations are used: (1) an aminoglycoside plus vancomycin, (2) an amino-glycoside plus a semisynthetic penicillin (nafcillin or methicillin), and (3) an aminoglycoside plus ceftazidime. In our experience, resolution of the infection occurs in approximately 75%–80% of the documented cases. However, *recurrent infection* following appropriate therapy or *early relapse* are absolute indications to remove the central line!

The metabolic complications include electrolyte imbalances (hyponatremia, hypernatremia, nonketotic hyperosmolar hyperglycemia, hypoglycemia, hypophosphatemia), trace metal deficiencies (zinc, copper, selenium, etc.), and abnormal liver function tests.

The preceding *caveats* have been emphasized by many authors, yet in carefully selected patients, *the complications resulting from central venous cannulation are minimized if the procedure is carried out by an experienced operator.* One must use meticulous, aseptic technique and closely monitor the patient for volume status, electrolytes, acid-base balance, and for regulation of blood sugar levels to an acceptable range of 120 mg to 180 mg/dl. **Note:** For patients on mechanical ventilators, the risk of pneumothorax is reduced by disconnecting the ventilator and mechanically ventilating the patient with a resuscitation bag (plus supplemental O_2) while the line is being inserted.

MANAGEMENT OF FLUID, ELECTROLYTE, AND METABOLIC PROBLEMS

Fluid Balance. Strict attention must be paid to the patient's daily intake, output, and body weight. To cover insensible losses, intake of fluids should exceed output by 500–800 ml/day except when the patient is receiving humidification via mechanical ventilation. Retention of body water or overhydration can hide actual weight loss due to depletion of fat and non-fatty tissue. When fluid restriction is necessary for volume overload, one may temporarily give (until status improves) 1.0 L/day of a concentrated TPN solution that contains 70 g of PRO (700 ml of 10% amino acid) and 210 g of CHO (300 ml of 70% dextrose) = 994 (280 + 714) kcal/day. See page 121 for fluid requirements.

Chemical Balance. Electrolyte and metabolic complications during TPN include hyponatremia, hypernatremia, nonketotic hyperosmolar hyperglycemia, hypoglycemia, hypophosphatemia, hypokalemia, hypocalcemia, hypomagnesemia, and acid-base disturbances. These problems are discussed below and elsewhere in the text (see p. 123). The key to preventing complications is close monitoring of the patient. When TPN is started, DeVault Jr. (*J Crit Illness* 4 [10]: 70–81, 1989) recommends that serum levels of electrolytes and phosphorus be measured twice daily, and that serum glucose concentrations be determined at least every 4 to 6 hours using a reagent strip. We utilize a ChemStrip® on fresh capillary blood obtained by finger stick. Then semiquantitative determinations are carried out with an Accu-Check® Blood Glucose Monitor. Initially, other tests (done daily) include serum calcium, serum magnesium, BUN, and creatinine. Later, when the patient's condition stabilizes, the preceding blood chemistry tests can be performed two to three times weekly. In more chronic situations, especially during prolonged TPN, one should be on the alert for fatty infiltration of the liver (cholestatic hyperbilirubinemia), loss of visceral protein, and trace metal deficiencies.

Sodium/Chloride. Usually enteral and TPN solutions with additives (see p. 97) provide adequate electrolytes. Nevertheless, the patient's electrolyte levels must be closely monitored! As a rule, sodium (Na) and chloride (Cl) are given in doses of about 60–180 mEq total/day; however, requirements may change rapidly in dynamic situations (see hypernatremia and hyponatremia below).

Hypernatremia. The reader is referred to a well-written, informative monograph titled "Nutrients in Enteral Feeding" (published by Ross Medical Laboratories, Columbus, OH, June 1989, pp. 35–36) that reviews hypernatremia and hyponatremia. *Relating to hypernatremia, a number of important points are made:*

(1) The common causes of high serum Na are dehydration, sweating, fever, excess solute load (from concentrated tube feedings high in protein), osmotic diuresis (polyuria associated with diabetes), head trauma, brain tumor, and cranial surgery (ADH deficiency).

(2) There may be little or no correlation between serum Na concentration and total body Na.

(3) Serum Na in excess of **170 mEq/L** constitutes a medical emergency; however, the hypernatremia must be corrected by water intake slowly in order to avoid cerebral edema.

(4) When hypernatremia occurs along with hyperglycemia in a patient being tube fed, one must consider the likelihood of hyperosmolar hyperglycemic nonketotic dehydration, referred to as the *tube feeding syndrome.* Immediate corrective action is necessary or death may result. The physiopathology and management of this syndrome has been described in detail by Bivins et al.[150]

Hyponatremia. Low serum sodium is a common finding in patients who are overhydrated, on diuretics, being tube fed, or are receiving TPN. Included in the differential diagnosis is the syndrome of inappropriate antidiuretic hormone (SIADH). Also one must rule out a laboratory error, a false result (seen in hyperlipidemia, high serum protein levels, hyperglycemia), or a dilutional hyponatremia associated with a low urinary sodium concentration less than 5 mEq/L (seen in congestive heart failure, cirrhosis, edema, ascites, hypoalbuminemia, and decreased total body K). Usually patients tolerate hyponatremia without major problems except when the serum Na concentration falls below **120 mEq/L,** at which point lethargy, coma, and seizures may occur. In this instance, IV hypertonic saline is given with caution. Routinely, the range of sodium given daily to patients is 75–120 mEq/L of TPN solution.

Potassium. Low levels of serum potassium (below 3.5 mg/dl) readily develop in patients on TPN. Hypertonic glucose, via central vein catheter, and the administraiton of insulin cause potassium (K) to shift from intercellular to extracellular spaces. Usually K needs are around 60–100 mEq/day, but requirements may increase markedly (e.g., 100–150 mEq/day) when diuretics, vasopressors, or inotropic agents are given. Also K losses are significant in amphotericin-induced ATN (acute tubular necrosis of the kidney). If untreated, hypokalemia may produce cardiotoxicity (with tachyarrhythmias), renal toxicity, and may even contribute to the development of rhabdomyolysis. Either potassium chloride or potassium phosphate may be given, depending upon the serum phosphate level.

Calcium. Losses in calcium via the kidney and bowel are often seen in hypermetabolic, catabolic states. Also reductions in total body calcium occur secondary to mobilization of calcium from the bone. Since 50–60% of serum calcium is bound to protein, malnourished patients with hypoalbuminemia may have spuriously low calcium

levels. To correct this error, the following formula may be used:
Corrected serum calcium = patient's serum calcium + [(4.0 − serum albumin) × (0.8)].

Phosphorus. See page 32.

Magnesium. See page 33.

Acid-Base Balance. Metabolic status must be followed closely with careful control of fluid and electrolyte balance. To manage metabolic **acidosis,** additional acetate* may be used to buffer the amino acid solutions used in TPN, or if acidosis is severe then bicarbonate is administered separately from the TPN solution. Therapy of metabolic **alkalosis** (a common disorder) consists of infusion of 0.9% NaCl solution, KCl (given orally if not urgently needed), and either a histamine H_2 receptor antagonist (e.g., cimetidine) or a carbonic anhydrase inhibitor such as acetazolamide (Friedman BS, Lumb PD: *J Intensive Care Med,* 5 [Suppl]: S22–S27, 1990). Also calcium chloride can be used (in tube feedings) to treat patients with mild to moderate hypochloremic alkalosis. Severe metabolic alkalosis justifies using IV dilute HCl (0.2 N) via a central vein catheter. See p. 123 and Table 16 (p. 124) regarding drug-nutrient problems.

PARENTERAL FORMULAS/INFUSIONS
ENERGY SOURCES

Table 15 shows the caloric density of the venous nutrient substrates. **As a source of energy, glucose (dextrose in water) will supply 3.4 kcal/g, protein (amino acids) 4.0 kcal/g, and fat 11 kcal/g (10% lipid emulsion) or 10 kcal/g (20% lipid emulsion).** Note the difference in energy conversion factors for CHO when given intravenously rather than by gut. Hydrated dextrose (dextrose monohydrate) has only 3.4 kcal/g, compared to anhydrous glucose which has a caloric yield of 4 kcal/g. Also observe that the manufactured fat infusions contain glycerol (to give tonicity) and egg yolk phospholipids (to act as an emulsifier), which add a small amount of CHO and FAT Calories respectively. Thus, 10% fat emulsion supplies 1.1 kcal/ml, and 20% emulsion supplies 2.0 kcal/ml.

FORMULA CONCENTRATIONS

The manufactured formulas for parenteral feeding vary in their concentrations: (1) *glucose* (dextrose 10% to 70%), (2) *amino acid* 3%

---

*The end product of acetate metabolism is bicarbonate.

Feeding the Patient

Table 15. CALORIC DENSITY OF VENOUS NUTRIENT SUBSTRATES

	g/L	Caloric Yield	kcal/L	kcal/ml
Dextrose 5%	50	3.4	170	0.17
Dextrose 10%	100	3.4	340	0.34
Dextrose 20%	200	3.4	680	0.65
Dextrose 30%	300	3.4	1020	1.02
Dextrose 40%	400	3.4	1360	1.36
Dextrose 50%	500	3.4	1700	1.70
Dextrose 60%	600	3.4	2040	2.04
Dextrose 70%	700	3.4	2380	2.38
Amino acids 3.5%	35	4.0	140	0.14
Amino acids 5.0%	50	4.0	200	0.20
Amino acids 8.5%	85	4.0	340	0.34
Amino acids 10%	100	4.0	400	0.40

Fat Emulsion 10%:
Soybean/safflower oil: 10 gm/100 ml × 9 kcal/g	=	90 kcal/dl
Egg yolk phospholipids: 1.2 g/100 ml × 9 kcal/g	=	11 kcal/dl
Glycerin: 2.25–2.5 g/100 ml × 4 kcal/g	=	9–10 kcal/dl
Total	=	110–111 kcal/dl
	=	1.1 kcal/ml

Fat Emulsion 20%:
Soybean/safflower oil: 20 gm/100 ml × 9 kcal/g	=	180 kcal/dl
Egg yolk phospholipids: 1.2 g/100 ml × 9 kcal/g	=	11 kcal/dl
Glycerin: 2.25–2.5 g/100 ml × 4 kcal/g	=	9–10 kcal/dl
Total	=	200–201 kcal/dl
	=	2.0 kcal/ml

to 10%, with or without electrolytes, and (3) **lipid emulsion** 10% and 20%. Solutions high in osmolarity will rapidly produce vein irritation and thrombophlebitis. As previously discussed, the peripheral venous system will not tolerate an infusate (PRO-CHO mixture) which has concentrations of amino acids higher than 4.25% and dextrose concentrations higher than 7.5 to 10% in the final mixture. *On the other hand, hypertonic solutions are well tolerated when given by central vein because of significant dilution from the ample flow of blood through the vena cava.* Lipid emulsions, both 10% and 20%, are isotonic (by the addition of glycerol) and may be infused peripherally without injury to the vein.

NUTRIENT REQUIREMENTS, INFUSION RATES[19,139]

The patient's tolerance for fluids and glucose load should be checked by starting parenteral feeding with 1 liter of formula on the first day, then continuing with 2 liters on the second day (providing there are no electrolyte or metabolic problems), and, if indicated, 3 liters on the third and succeeding days. A continuous infusion rate of 125 ml/hr (barely over 2 ml/min) will provide 3 L/24 hrs. Patients without cardiac, renal, or pulmonary disease usually will tolerate 3 liters of fluid daily. *Dextrose tolerance* may be checked by providing the estimated daily fluid intake while advancing the strength of the dextrose solution via TPN, for example, $D_{10} \rightarrow D_{20} \rightarrow D_{25} \rightarrow D_{30}$. This approach guarantees appropriate intake of fluids while determining the patient's ability to handle a glucose load.

THE NUTRIENT REQUIREMENTS AND INFUSION RATES FOR THE SUBSTRATES ARE AS FOLLOWS:

(1) Carbohydrate (CHO). Sufficient glucose (not excessive amounts) should be given to obtain a maximal protein-sparing effect and to supply the requirements of glucose dependent tissue, including the brain, red and white blood cells, bone marrow, peripheral nerves, and renal medulla. Initially, glucose is given at a dosage of around 200 g/day to check the patient's tolerance. *To help avoid hyperglycemia Wolfe and colleagues recommended that the* **optimal rate** *of delivering glucose (dextrose) intravenously in the stressed patient should be no more than 0.3 g/kg/hr (5 mg/kg/min).*[151]

The undesirable consequences of high glucose loads are[77,152-154] (1) lipogenesis, (2) fatty liver, (3) hyperosmolar nonketotic coma, (4) inordinate production of carbon dioxide with a high RQ, and (5) excessive ventilatory drive. Furthermore, unreasonably large amounts of CHO can precipitate acute respiratory failure in patients with COPD (chronic obstructive pulmonary disease) and impair weaning in ventilator-dependent patients. Finally, correction of nutritional deficits will aid weaning of malnourished, ventilator-dependent patients (Larca L, Greenbaum DM: *Crit Care Med* 10: 297–300, 1982).

Persistent hyperglycemia requires treatment with insulin. An excellent approach is to give regular insulin (RI) subcutaneously. Starting with 3 units of RI for a blood sugar level of 200–250 mg/dl, the dose is increased by 3 units for every 50 mg/dl rise in blood sugar above 250 mg/dl. Thus, at a level of 350–400 mg/dl, the dose of RI is 12 units. Because of its short action, adjusted doses of RI are given every 4 to 6 hours. The addition of insulin to the TPN bag presents problems because of insulin binding which occurs to the bag and PVC tubing. We

Feeding the Patient

do not advocate this approach. *The late development of hyperglycemia in a stable patient often is a harbinger of a new infection or complication.*[155] Also, although uncommon, one should consider the possibility of a *chromium deficiency* (p. 100) when glucose intolerance is encountered. **Note:** Testing for urinary glucose on patients receiving TPN is of little or no use ... blood levels must be determined!

(2) Protein (PRO). The amount of nitrogen (amino acids) administered should not only be enough to maintain visceral protein but also replenish nitrogen deficit by putting the patient in a ***positive nitrogen balance.*** Ideal values of N balance range from +1 to +4 g/24 hrs[36]; however, higher values from +4 to +6 are customary goals for patients with significant protein depletion.[19] Although liberal amounts of crystalline amino acid solutions can be given to patients without renal or hepatic failure, *the zealous overfeeding of protein should be guarded against since excessive intake can increase ventilatory drive.*[156] Routinely, protein goals can be achieved by providing between 1.0 g/kg/day of PRO (simple starvation) to as high as 2.5 g/kg/day (severe burns or late sepsis) as shown in Table 13, page 39. As a general rule, critically ill patients under considerable stress are given PRO in the range of 1.5 to 2.0 g/kg/day. However, for chronic renal failure patients who are not on dialysis, restriction of PRO intake is recommended (e.g., 0.55 g/kg/day) with 50% of the PRO being of high biologic value. For those adults being treated with *hemodialysis,* PRO intake should be in the range of 1.0–1.2 g/kg/day. For ambulatory patients on *peritoneal dialysis,* PRO intake is increased to 1.2–1.5 g/kg/day because of the large losses of PRO in each dialysate.
Note: gms PRO/6.25 = gms Nitrogen (N).

Branched-chain amino acids (BCAAs) may be useful in the dietary management of patients with moderate to severe hepatic encephalopathy or renal failure. In this group of patients, PRO intake usually is restricted to 40–70 g/day. Enriched solutions are utilized that contain the essential amino acids *leucine, isoleucine, and valine* (BCAAs) + other essential and nonessential amino acids + electrolytes. The BCAAs are oxidized in skeletal muscle (also in fatty tissue) and have the advantage of increasing hepatic protein synthesis, improving nitrogen balance, and lowering skeletal muscle turnover (presumably reduced catabolism). Conventional formulas are routinely given if the encephalopathy is mild or the BUN has stabilized below 100 mg/dl.[142] At the University of Iowa Hospitals and Clinics we rarely use specialty TPN products in renal disease except in acute tubular necrosis.

(3) Fat (FAT).[19,36,139] In TPN, fat is administered intravenously as polyunsaturated, long-chain triglycerides (LCTs) derived from soybean and/or safflower oils. As discussed on p.p. 91, 92, the lipid emulsion is available in 10% and 20% (wt/vol) concentrations. Catabolic, malnourished patients can readily utilize 1–2 g/kg/day of lipid emulsion, and higher amounts have been given (up to 4 g/kg/day) without unfavorable results. *The present recommendation is that fat not exceed 50%–60% of the patient's total energy intake (measured as kcal/day) so that reticuloendothelial dysfunction will not occur.*

The goal is to avoid hyperlipidemia, thus the *rate of the infusion* (slow vs fast) becomes important. In adults, the initial infusion rate for **10%** lipid is 1 ml/min. After 30 minutes, if no untoward reactions occur, the rate may be increased but not exceed 100 ml/hour. Care is taken that only 500 ml are given the first day; subsequently, the daily dosage should not exceed 2.5 g/kg body weight. For the **20%** lipid emulsion, the intravenous rates are half those of the 10% emulsion.

It appears that a *slow infusion* of fat emulsion over 16–20 hours may be preferable to a *rapid delivery* over 6–8 hours.[157] When slow feedings are administered to nonstressed patients, the triglyceride levels peak 4–6 hours after the infusion is started and then plateau during the next 8–10 hours before falling to pretreatment levels. When slow infusions are given to stressed patients, the triglyceride levels usually climb until the end of the feeding before declining. However, with fast infusions in stressed patients, the triglyceride levels may rise precipitously and then decline slowly until Km (Michaelis constant) is reached; thereafter the fall is appropriate. Ergo, fat emulsions are given slowly at the University of Iowa Hospitals and Clinics over 16–20 hours (e.g., 50–60 ml/hr for 1000 ml of a 10% emulsion). When the slow infusion of fat is used, triglyceride levels may be checked anytime (during and/or after the IV feeding) but blood samples must not be drawn from the IV line since fat residue would give a falsely high triglyceride value and effect other laboratory tests. We conservatively aim for triglyceride levels under 150 mg/dl in the unstressed patient and under 250 mg/dl in the stressed patient.[158] It is not uncommon for the reticuloendothelial system to begin phagocytosis of fat when triglyceride levels are above 150 mg/dl. If fast delivery of fat is employed, then a triglyceride sample is taken 6 to 8 hours after the infusion. **Note:** Stressed patients may lack adequate tissue *carnitine* activity. Since carnitine is required to shuttle LCTs across the mitochondrial membranes for subsequent oxidation and energy availability, a drop in carnitine activity may predispose to FFA accumulation, especially with increased rates of IV fat infusions.

The addition of fat (lipid) emulsion to a parenteral feeding program of amino acids + glucose has several distinct advantages.[19,27,36,137,159] Lipid emulsions (LCTs) are isotonic, can be given per peripheral vein without damaging the endothelium of the vessel, provide essential fatty acids *(linoleic, linolenic, and arachidonic)*, are a major source of calories in a relatively small volume of solution, have a nitrogen-sparing effect (although not as much as (CHO), yield less CO_2 than combustion of either CHO or PRO,[160] do not require insulin, do not cause a fatty liver, do not stimulate the pancreas when given intravenously (important in pancreatitis and biliary dysfunction), and do not block the immune response. In addition, increasing the proportion of fat calories and decreasing CHO calories will lower CO_2 production and RQ, thus reducing ventilatory requirements.

Regarding lipids, there are several important forewarnings. (1) FAT is a major source of calories in hypermetabolic stress but is *not* used in shock or late sepsis other than to supply the necessary essential fatty acids (EFAs). Routinely we give 500 ml of 10% fat emulsion intravenously two or three times a week to maintain adequate serum and tissue levels of *linoleic acid.* (2) Even patients with hyperlipidemia or liver disease require some fat emulsion (LCTs) to prevent EFA deficiency. (3) To be safe, one should *not* start IV lipids without obtaining a baseline triglyceride level. Then if the fat emulsion is given, the patient's serum triglyceride value should be determined again before the next infusion. Since fat emulsion is cleared by the enzyme *lipoprotein lipase,* the infusion rate vs clearance rate becomes an important factor. Therefore, if a lipid emulsion is given in a relatively short period of time, a reasonable procedure is to wait 6 to 8 hours after the infusion has finished before drawing a blood sample. In extended TPN, if there are no initial problems in lipid clearance, the serum triglyceride level can be rechecked twice a week as indicated.

Medium-chain triglycerides (MCTs). Concern regarding the potential harmful effects of long-chain triglyceride infusions has spurred the *enteral use* of medium-chain triglycerides (MCTs) as an alternate source of fat, especially when gut absorption is compromised. MCTs are derived from fractionated coconut oil and contain fatty acid molecules that have chain lengths of 6 to 12 carbon atoms. Unlike LCTs, medium-chain fats are not formed into chylomicrons and, by bypassing the lymphatic route, they do not interfere with the function of the reticuloendothelial system. Furthermore, the component fatty acids of MCTs are transported as free fatty acids attached to albumin (without esterification) directly to the liver via the portal vein, and they provide better N balance than LCTs.[161] *A noteworthy bit of information: MCTs lack linoleic acid (an essential fatty acid) and therefore cannot be used as the sole source of fat in the diet.* Instead, safflower or soybean oil (LCTs) must be added in order to provide linoleic acid.

Fact: Essential fatty acids (EFAs) are necessary for synthesis of normal cell membranes. At least 2-3% of the patient's total caloric intake should consist of linoleic acid to avoid EFA deficiency.[162] Liposyn II 10% and 20% (Abbott Laboratories) has an equal mixture of safflower oil and soybean oil as its fatty acid source and contains 65.8% linoleic acid. All other marketed IV fat emulsion products* have only soybean oil and contain 49-60% linoleic acid.

MCTs are ideal as a fat supplement in patients with malabsorption of the small bowel, blind loop syndrome, sprue, celiac disease, radiation enteritis, chronic liver disease, and fat-induced hyperlipidemia. MCTs also can be utilized effectively and safely in patients with pancreatic insufficiency, since large amounts of these lipids are hydrolyzed in the stomach and small intestine without the enzyme *pancreatic lipase*. Because of high intraluminal osmolality, MCTs must be given *slowly* to avoid gastric upset, cramps, and diarrhea.

ADDITIVES

Electrolytes. Commercially available amino acid solutions with electrolytes supply the basic requirements (except calcium) for most patients and include sodium, potassium, chloride, magnesium, acetate, and phosphate. To augment electrolyte-containing amino acid solutions, additives include sodium chloride, sodium acetate, sodium phosphates, potassium chloride, potassium acetate, potassium phosphates, magnesium sulfate, calcium gluconate and calcium chloride. In unusual circumstances, amino acid preparations *without electrolytes* are necessary. These solutions provide only chloride and acetate with minimal to no sodium or phosphate. Electrolyte additives are used then to build a solution more appropriate for the patient (e.g., low phosphate and low magnesium in renal dysfunction). It is important to note, however, that sodium, potassium, calcium magnesium, and phosphorus may be critical in anabolism. The daily requirements for these electrolytes in pro-

---

*Fat emulsion marketing companies: Intralipid = Clintec Nutrition Co.; Liposyn = Abbott Laboratories; NutriLipid = Kendall McGaw Laboratories; Soyacal = Alpha Therapeutic Corp.

tein-calorie malnutrition are as follows: sodium 80–180 mEq, potassium 70–150 mEq, calcium 10–22 mEq, magnesium 8–24 mEq, and phosphorus 10–40 mmol (DeVault Jr: *J Crit Illness* 4 [10]: 57, 1989.

Vitamins. A vital role is played by vitamins as enzyme cofactors in many metabolic pathways. The clinical manifestations of fat- and water-soluble vitamin deficiencies are discussed on page 112. For daily multivitamin maintenance while on TPN, either Berocca Parenteral Nutrition (Roche Labs) or M.V.I.-12 (Rorer Pharmaceuticals) may be given. Both preparations contain similar amounts of water-soluble and oil-soluble vitamins as shown below:

VITAMIN CONTENT OF BEROCCA PARENTERAL NUTRITION AND M.V.I.-12
(for adults and children above age 11)

Vitamin	Content
Vitamin A (retinol)	3300 USP (1 mg)
Vitamin B_1 (thiamine HCl)	3 mg
Vitamin B_2 (riboflavin)	3.6 mg
Niacinamide	40 mg
Vitamin B_6 (pyridoxine HCl)	4 mg
Vitamin B_{12} (cyanocobalamin)	5 µg*
Vitamin C (ascorbic acid)	100 mg**
Vitamin D (ergocalciferol)	200 USP units (5 µg)
Vitamin E (dl-alpha tocopherol)	10 USP units (10 mg)
Folic acid	400 µg
Niacinamide	40 mg
d-Biotin	60 µg
Dexpanthenol (pantothenic acid)	15 mg

*B_{12} deficiency is highly unlikely in malnourished patients unless they have pernicious anemia or chronic malabsorption.

**Supplemental vitamin C (300–500 mg/day) has been recommended for hypermetabolic patients receiving TPN.

Note: A daily dosage of 2 ml (2 vials of 1 ml each) of Berocca Parenteral Nutrition and 10 ml (2 vials of 5 ml each) of M.V.I.-12 will provide the above vitamins at levels recommended by the Nutrition Advisory Group, American Medical Association, Department of Foods and Nutrition, 1975 (JPEN 3: 258–269, Jul–Aug 1979). Usually the vitamin concentrate is ordered by the physician on a daily or as-needed basis and added to standard TPN formulations. Observe that vitamin K is absent from the above multivitamin infusions. Thus, vitamin K, 10 mg (AquaMephyton, Merck Sharp & Dohme), is administered intramuscularly once a week, except when the patient is on anti-coagulant therapy.

Heparin/Insulin. Because of the very low incidence of major vein thrombosis at our hospital, we do not routinely add heparin to the TPN solution for this specific purpose. Heparin, however, may be added to the fat emulsion bottle (to activate lipoprotein lipase) at a concentration of 1–2 units/ml prior to administration. The addition of insulin for persistent hyperglycemia is discussed on page 93.

Minerals/Trace Metals. Under normal conditions, only 100–200 mg of calcium is absorbed daily from the intestine. During TPN, our policy is to add two ampules (10 ml each) of *calcium gluconate* (4.6 mEq/10 ml) daily for a total dose of 186 mg calcium/day. *Iron* is infrequently required. When indicated, iron dextran (for IV use) may be given up to 100 ml/L of TPN solution but ***only*** upon definite demonstration of iron deficiency anemia; a test dose is recommended to prevent severe allergic reactions. Rarely is *iodine* supplementation needed. *Trace metal deficiencies* are uncommon in short-term TPN but do occur in patients on extended (longer than 3–4 weeks) TPN. The essential trace elements include zinc, copper, manganese, selenium, molybdenum, and chromium. The recommended daily intravenous doses (for adults) are listed on the next page, followed by a short discussion of the clinical manifestations of trace metal deficiencies. With the exception of molybdenum, the trace metals (Zn, Cu, Mn, Se, and Cr) are supplied in a product that is marketed as *Multitrace 5* (Armour); 1 ml of Multitrace may be administered in one bottle of TPN solution daily (higher doses are given for intestinal losses and repletion).

Zinc serves as a cofactor for more than 70 different enzymes and is essential for promoting wound healing and a positive nitrogen balance. Zinc deficiency may be manifested as a dermatitis that can be confused with the dermatitis of essential fatty acid deficiency.

RECOMMENDED DAILY IV DOSES (FOR ADULTS) OF THE ESSENTIAL TRACE ELEMENTS*

NAME	DOSAGE
Zinc	2.5–4.0 mg (+2 mg in catabolic state; +17.1 mg/L of stool or ileostomy output)
Copper	0.5–1.5 mg
Manganese	0.15–0.8 mg
Selenium	50–200 µg (100 µg/d for repletion)
Molybdenum	150–500 µg (300–500 µg/d for repletion)
Chromium	10–15 µg (20 µg/d with intestinal losses; 150 µg/d for repletion)

*RDAs (American Medical Association, Department of Foods and Nutrition: JAMA 241: 2051–2054, 1979; also reference 19, pp. 16, 17)

Hypomagnesemia may go unrecognized until symptoms develop that resemble those seen in hypocalcemia, namely jerky and involuntary movements, twitching, convulsions, and mental confusion. See pages 32, 33 for a detailed discussion of serum magnesium and phosphorus. *Copper* is a component of at least 16 metalloproteins. Deficiency in this trace element may result in anemia, neutropenia, thrombocytopenia, impaired humoral immunity, pigment changes, and ataxia (DeVault Jr: *J Crit Illness* 4 (9): 75–94, 1989). *Manganese* serves as a cofactor for many enzyme systems. Manganese deficiency (extremely rare) is characterized by hypercholesterolemia, impaired gluconeogenesis, bone and connective tissue deformities, and prolongation of the prothrombin time (Jeejeebhoy KN *in* Shoemaker WC et al (eds): *Textbook of Critical Care,* ed. 2. Philadelphia, WB Saunders, 1989, pp. 1093–1118). *Selenium* is distributed throughout the body and is thought to protect cells from damage due to oxygen free radicals (superoxide, peroxide, hydrolyl radicals). *Chromium deficiency* has been associated with glucose intolerance (primarily from insulin resistance) and neuropathy.[163] The RQ declines since glucose cannot be metabolized efficiently. Rather recently a *molybdenum-deficient* patient on TPN developed an amino acid intolerance that was corrected by the addition of molybdenum.[164] Informative references on the essential vitamins and trace minerals are listed on page 34, at the end of the section marked "Miscellaneous." **Note:** Do not give zinc or chromium in the presence of renal dysfunction. Also, copper and manganese should be avoided in patients with biliary tract obstruction or severe liver dysfunction. To do otherwise may rapidly result in toxicity because the normal avenues of excretion for these trace metals would be blocked!

SOLUTIONS, TECHNIQUES, PROCEDURES

In the parenteral administration of nutrition, there are important common denominators; however, technical and procedural modifications often are found between hospitals. For example, the TPN formulas used at our medical center are made up of amino acids + dextrose in one container (see mixing techniques below), and the fat emulsion remains (as manufactured) in a separate bottle. Both solutions are given simultaneously via a Y connector to a common line, with the option of an in-line filter on the side of the amino acid + dextrose solution. In sharp contrast to this method of delivering TPN, Jensen and Bistrian[144] prepare a stock solution of lipid emulsion (10% to 20%), amino acids (10%), and dextrose (70%) in a single 24-hour container at selected concentrations in a given volume. First the lipid is mixed with the amino acid solution, then the dextrose solution is added, followed by electrolytes, vitamins, and trace elements. This method of preparation and administration has been termed "total-nutrient-admixture" or the "3-in-1" system. While the system is simple and may reduce costs, it is applicable only for *the stable patient.* Use of this admixture in the critically ill population (i.e., *the unstable patient*) may increase waste and costs if frequent electrolyte changes are necessary.[165] **Note:** Many medications and chemotherapeutic agents are incompatible with TPN solutions and must be given separately.

THE STANDARD PARENTERAL FEEDING PROGRAM AT THE UNIVERSITY OF IOWA HOSPITALS AND CLINICS IS AS FOLLOWS:

(1) **For peripheral venous nutrition (PVN).** The infusion employed consists of 4.25% amino acid with electrolytes and 10% dextrose. The pharmacist prepares this stock solution by mixing 500 ml of 8.5% amino acid and 500 ml of 20% dextrose in water, using strictly sterile technique under a laminar flow hood. A high-speed **computerized compounder** provides fast, accurate mixing. The TPN infusion is given over 24 hours in a peripheral vein at a predetermined rate, but usually not faster than 90 ml/hr (2160 ml/24 hrs). In addition, 500–1000 ml of a 10% fat emulsion or 500 ml of a 20% fat emulsion is administered 16–20 hours daily* (or 2–3

---

*Biochemical tests are obtained before starting the next infusion of fat.

Feeding the Patient

times/week to prevent EFA deficiency), as discussed on page 97. If 500 ml of 20% fat emulsion is given daily along with the amino acid + dextrose solution, then the maximal total calories supplied by all of the nutrients = 2101 kcal/day, and the total volume = 2.660 L/day (2.160 L + 0.5 L):

CHO: $100 \text{ g/L} \times 3.4 \text{ kcal/g} = 340 \text{ kcal/L} \times 2.160 \text{ L} = 734.4 \text{ kcal}$

PRO: $42.5 \text{ g/L} \times 4.0 \text{ kcal/g} = 170 \text{ kcal/L} \times 2.160 \text{ L} = 367.2 \text{ kcal}$

FAT: $200 \text{ g/L} \times 10 \text{ kcal/g} = 2000 \text{ kcal/L} \times \underline{0.500} \text{ L} = \underline{1000.0} \text{ kcal}$

$\qquad\qquad\qquad\qquad\qquad\qquad\qquad\quad$ 2.660 L/day 2101.6 kcal/day

(2) **For total parenteral nutrition (TPN),** a standard solution for general use (suitable in many cases) is prepared by mixing 500 ml of 8.5% amino acids + electrolytes with 500 ml of 50% dextrose in water (D_{50}). The final solution will consist of 4.25% amino acids and 25% dextrose and will have a caloric value of about 1.0 kcal/ml and a NPC:nitrogen ratio of approximately 125:1. As a general rule, the infusion is given continuously in the superior vena cava at a rate of 90 ml/hr. The routine for adding IV lipids is the same as described above. When clinically indicated, the standard formula can be modified by changing the proportions of the amino acids and dextrose solutions. For example, the amount of CHO (dextrose) calories can be reduced relative to the PRO (amino acid) calories by adding 200 ml of sterile water to 300 ml of 50% dextrose. When this diluted dextrose solution (500 ml of D_{30}) is mixed with 500 ml of 8.5% amino acids, the final solution will consist of 1.0 liter of 4.25% amino acids and 15% dextrose. In a similar fashion, the same method may be used to change the final concentration of amino acids.

(3) **For cycled TPN at home,** the patient is first given a trial on nocturnal TPN while in the hospital. Usually a period of 1–2 weeks is required for the patient and/or a member of the family to learn how to properly handle all of the paraphernalia and to take care of the silastic catheter. To be successful, home TPN requires commitment of the patient (or helper) to learn new skills and to follow instructions of the TPN nurse. Otherwise, failure will surely result!

Our routine[166] is to start the patient's infusion rate at about 90 ml/hr for the first hour, then to step up the rate to 180 ml/hr for the next 10± hours, and subsequently slow the infusion back down to 90 ml/hr for the last hour or so. Even slower initial and termination rates are used if hyperglycemia or rebound hypoglycemia should occur. During the daytime the venous access port is plugged (Luer-Loc cap) and flushed with heparin. In selected patients, low-dose coumadin (1 mg/day) *per os* is employed to reduce the risk of venous thrombosis.[167]

One important requirement is to *closely monitor* the patient's blood sugar, electrolytes, and liver enzymes. After the patient has reached a stable state on cyclic, nocturnal TPN, the physician writes a prescription for the composition of the TPN solution plus additives (delivered to the health care company supplying the formula), and the patient is discharged home. A return appointment is made for every 2 ± weeks to check on the patient's weight, fluid balance, and blood chemistry values. Later, if all goes well, follow-up appointments are made for every 4–6 weeks. **Note:** Cycled TPN in the patient's home may have distinct advantages over continuous infusion but *should not be used on insulin-dependent patients.*

(4) **For administering TPN solutions,** *volumetric infusion devices, known as pumps, have been a great help in achieving reliable infusion rates.* These devices must be kept clean; they should be wiped daily with alcohol and promptly cleaned if solutions are spilled on them. Any malfunction of the pump should be reported immediately. During operation, the pump cord always is kept plugged into the electric outlet, but the pump itself must be shut off if there is air in the TPN tubing or any disruption in the line. Instructions on operating and cleaning the infusion pumps are furnished by the manufacturers.

CALCULATING PARENTERAL FEEDINGS

Steps in Preparing Formulas for Parenteral Nutrition

STEP 1. Measure the patient's total energy requirement (kcal/day) by indirect calorimetry. Use the Harris-Benedict formula with correction factors if a metabolic cart is not available.

STEP 2. Determine the daily fluid requirement. Restrict fluids and/or sodium as needed.

STEP 3. Estimate the PRO (amino acid) requirement from the figures shown in STEP 4 below or from Table 13, page 39. The objective is to maintain visceral protein and to replenish N (nitrogen) deficits.

Feeding the Patient

STEP 4. Calculate the nonprotein Calories: multiply the grams of PRO (STEP 3) × 4 to obtain the total kcal of PRO/day, then subtract the kcal of PRO from the total Calories (STEP 1). The nonprotein Calories (dextrose and lipid) are expressed as a ratio of CHO to FAT (CHO/FAT) or separately as a percentage of the total energy requirement that includes PRO. *The substrate requirements are shown below according to the levels of stress:*[36]

STRESS LEVEL:	NONE (Starvation)	MODERATE (Poly trauma)	EARLY SEVERE	LATE SEVERE
NPC:N (kcal/gN)	150:1	100:1	100:1	80:1
PRO needs (g/kg/d)	1	1.5	2	2–2.5
Amino acids(%)	15	20	25	30
FAT (%)	25	30	35	EFA*
CHO (%)	60	50	40	70
NPC:CHO/FAT (ratio, %)	70/30	60/40	50/50	100/EFA*

EFA = Essential fatty acids are not only necessary but also tolerated.

NOTE: See Table 13, page 39.

STEP 5. To calculate the grams of dextrose, divide the total CHO calories by 3.4. See step 9 to calculate the strength (%) of the dextrose solution. **Note:** The optimal rate of administering IV glucose in the stressed patient is 3–5 mg/kg/min, but not more than 5 mg/kg/min.

STEP 6. To calculate the volume of FAT (lipid emulsion) required, divide the total FAT Calories by 2 if a 20% fat emulsion is used. **Note:** 20% lipids = 2.0 kcal/ml, and 10% lipids = 1.1 kcal/ml.

STEP 7. Electrolytes, vitamins, and minerals are added for maintenance and replenishment.

STEP 8. Nitrogen balance and serum triglyceride clearance are determined to assess adequacy of PRO (amino acid) and FAT (lipid) infusions. Avoid overfeeding of protein. *For* *maintenance,* provide enough PRO so that N intake equals N output. *For repletion,* achieve a positive N balance.

STEP 9. The strength (%) of the solutions administered for TPN depends upon the patient's daily CHO, PRO, FAT, and fluid requirements. For example, to calculate the % of dextrose solution needed, subtract the volume (ml) of fat emulsion from the total volume of the daily infusion. Next, divide the amount of dextrose needed (g/day) by the volume (ml) of the nonfat solution.

NOTE: *Closely check the patient's status daily, including weight, fluid intake, and output. Also monitor the various appropriate laboratory tests as previously discussed in detail.*

Practical Applications

Using the above steps, let us now review how the TPN formula was calculated for the case study presented on pages 59–66. The patient was a 22-year-old, ventilator-dependent male (ht. 183 cm, wt. 70 kg) who had leukemia and a pulmonary fungal infection (cephalosporium). Anthropometric and laboratory data revealed significant depletion of his energy and protein stores (marasmus-kwashiorkor).

STEP 1. **Total Energy Need:** The patient's REE of 3274 kcal/day (obtained by indirect calorimetry) was multiplied by 1.1 (activity factor, p. 00) to give the final energy requirement of 3601 kcal/day.

STEP 2. **Maintenance Fluid Requirement:** Although mildly uremic, the patient tolerated 2800 ml of fluid/day without any difficulty.

STEP 3. **Protein Requirement:** Based on the high level of stress (see STRESS LEVEL, p. 104 and also Table 13, p. 39), the patient was given 1.7 g/kg/day of PRO, which in a 70 kg person calculates to 1.7 × 70 = 119 g PRO. In fact, 120 g PRO/day were given.

STEP 4. **Nonprotein Calories (NPC) and CHO/FAT Ratio:** First, the energy supplied by PRO (kcal/day) was obtained by multiplying 120 g PRO (see step 3) by its physiologic fuel value of 4.0 (e.g., 120 × 4.0 = 480 kcal/day). Then to calculate the NPCs, the Calories of PRO were subtracted from the total Calories (e.g., 3601 − 480 = 3121 nonprotein Calories). Next, a ratio of 50/50 was selected for the patient as being appropriate for his high degree of stress. Thus, each of the NPC substrates should provide 1560 Calories (3121 ÷ 2 = 1560). Actually, the patient received 1530 Calories of CHO and 1500 Calories of FAT daily, which is very close to the calculated 1560 Calories/day for CHO and FAT each and the 50/50 ratio.

STEP 5. **Carbohydrate Requirement:** Since the patient's CHO requirement was being met by IV dextrose and not oral glucose, the grams of CHO to be given were determined by dividing his total CHO Calories/day by the energy conversion factor for dextrose, which is 3.4. The calculation is as follows: 1530 ÷ 3.4 = 450 g CHO/day.

STEP 6. **Fat Requirement:** To deliver 150 g FAT/day and keep within the total fluid restraints (2800 ml/day), a 20% FAT emulsion was used instead of the 10% concentration. Since 20% lipids = 2 kcal/ml, the volume (ml) of lipid to be delivered is calculated by dividing FAT Calories by 2: 1500 ÷ 2 = 750 ml of lipid emulsion.

STEP 7. **Additives:** Electrolytes, vitamins, and minerals were added for maintenance and to replenish deficits (pp. 32, 33, 89–91, and 97–100.).

STEP 8. **Nitrogen Balance/Serum Triglyceride:** The nitrogen balance of the patient was determined to be +3.4 N/24 hrs, and the serum triglyceride level was 186 mg/dl (p. 65) after two weeks of nutritional therapy.

STEP 9. **Strength (%) of Nonfat Substrates:** To calculate the % of dextrose given the patient, subtract 750 ml (volume of 20% fat emulsion) from 2800 ml (volume of daily infusion): 2800 − 750 = 2050 ml. Next, divide 450 (g/day of dextrose) by 2050 (volume of nonfat solution): 450 ÷ 2050 = 0.2195 g CHO/1.0 ml = 21.9 g/100 ml = **21.9% dextrose.** To calculate the % of PRO (amino acids), divide the amount of PRO to be given (120 g/day) by 2050 ml (volume of nonfat solution): 120 ÷ 2050 = 0.058 g PRO/1.0 ml = 5.8 g/100 ml = **5.8% amino acids.**

Final Comment: To meet the above requirements, the following formulas were given: 1412 ml of 8.5% amino acids

+ 643 ml of 70% dextrose (in the same container), plus 750 ml of 20% lipid emulsion (in a separate bottle). The final volume of fluid was 2805 ml (2055 ml + 750 ml = 2805 ml). *Thus, the IV solutions supplied:* 480 Calories of PRO (120 g/day), 1530 Calories of dextrose (450 g CHO/day), and 1500 Calories of lipid emulsion (150 g FAT/day*). And if you wish to challenge your calculations skills further, one liter of amino acids + dextrose solution will contain 313 ml of 70% dextrose (D_{70}) and 687 ml of 8.5% amino acids. But the final concentration (as already determined above) will be 21.9% dextrose (313 × 70/1000) and 5.8% amino acids (687 × 8.5/1000). From a practical standpoint, dextrose solution is prescribed at our hospital in 2.5% to 5% increments. So in this particular case, the closest concentration of dextrose is 22.5%. **Note:** The above mixing procedure works best when the hospital pharmacy utilizes a *computerized compounder* to prepare the solutions. If the auto-mixing instrument is not available, then the final mls of amino acids and dextrose may be rounded to the nearest 50 ml.

Suggested Reading (Enteral/Parenteral feeding)

Dietary formulations for enteral and parenteral nutrition have been briefly reviewed in this chapter. For more detailed information, the following references are recommended:

(1) Bernard MA, Jacobs DO, Rombeau JL (eds): *Nutritional and Metabolic Support of Hospitalized Patients,* Philadelphia, WB Saunders Co, 1981.

(2) Grant JP: *Handbook of Total Parenteral Nutrition,* Philadelphia, WB Saunders Co, 1980.

(3) Heimburger DC, Weisner RL: Guidelines for evaluating and categorizing enteral feeding formulas according to therapeutic equivalence. *JPEN* 9: 61–67, 1985.

(4) Koruda MJ, Guenter P, Rombeau JL: Enteral nutrition in the critically ill. *Crit Care Clinics* 3 (1): 133–153, 1987.

(5) Lang CE (ed): *Nutritional Support in Critical Care,* Rockville, MD, Aspen Publishers, 1987.

*Actually, the amount of fat is slightly less because of the added glycerol.

(6) Maillet JO: Calculating parenteral feedings—A programmed instruction. *Am Dietetic Assn* 84 (11): 1312–1323, 1984.

(7) Rombeau JL, Caldwell MD (eds): *Enteral and Tube Feeding,* Philadelphia, WB Saunders Co, 1984.

(8) Rombeau JL, Caldwell MD (eds): *Parenteral Nutrition,* Philadelphia, WB Saunders Co, 1986.

(9) Silberman H, Eisenberg D: *Parenteral and Enteral Nutrition for the Hospitalized Patient,* Norwalk, CT, Appleton-Century-Crofts, 1987.

(10) Halpern SL (ed): *Quick Reference to Clinical Nutrition,* 2nd edition, Philadelphia, JB Lippincott Co, 1987.

(11) Blackburn GL, Bell SJ, Mullen JL (eds): *Nutritional Medicine; A Case Management Approach,* Philadelphia, WB Saunders Co, 1989.

MARKETING COMPANIES

The following list gives the names of the companies (in alphabetical order) that market nutritional products. The listing is for general information and is not intended to be complete. Each product is shown along with the appropriate manufacturing company and is specified as being for enteral or parenteral feeding.

Marketing Company / Product

Abbott Laboratories (Hospital Products Division)
Abbott Park
North Chicago, IL 60064

Parenteral: Aminosyn 3.5%, 5%, 7%, 8.5%, 10% (with and without electrolytes); Aminosyn HBC 7%; Aminosyn 3.5% M; Aminosyn pH 6.7%, 8.5%, 10% (with and without electrolytes); Aminosyn PF 7%, 10%; Aminosyn RF 5.2%; Aminosyn II 3.5%, 5%, 7%, 8.5%, 10% (with and without electrolytes); Aminosyn II 3.5%M. Cystein HCL. Liposyn II 10%, 20%; Liposyn III 10%, 20%. Micro-nutrient additives

Alpha Therapeutic Corp.
5555 Valley Boulevard
Los Angeles, CA 90032

Parenteral: Soyacal 10%, 20%.

Biosearch Medical Products, Inc.
P.O. Box 1700
35 Industrial Parkway
Somerville, NJ 08876

Enteral: Entri-Pac with Entrition.

Clintec Nutrition Co.
(Affiliate of Baxter Healthcare Corp.)
Deerfield, IL 60015

Parenteral: BranchAmin 4%, RenAmin 6.5%. Travasol 3.5%, 5.5%, 8.5%, 10% (with or without electrolytes). High concentrations of dextrose (10% to 70%). Micro-nutrient additives.
Enteral: Travasorb, Travasorb HN, Travasorb Hepatic, Travasorb Renal, Travasorb MCT.
NOTE: Clintec also markets KabiVitrum products, Carnation Instant Breakfast, and Carnation Peptamen.

KabiVitrum, Inc.
1311 Harbor Bay Parkway
Alameda, CA 94501

Parenteral: Intralipid 10%, 20%. Novamine 11.4%, 15%. Aminess 5.2%.
NOTE: KabiVitrum products are marketed by Clintec Nutrition Co.

Kendall McGaw Labs., Inc.
2525 McGaw Ave.
Irvine, CA 92714

Parenteral: FreAmine III (with electrolytes) 3%, 5%, 8.5%, 10%. FreAmine HBC 6.9%. HepatAmine 8%. NephrAmine 5.4%. NutriLipid 10%, 20%. ProcalAmine (3% AA and 3% Glycerin with electrolytes). TophAmine 6%, 10%.
Enteral: Amin-Aid. Hepatic-Aid II. Traum-Aid, Traum-Aid HBC. Ucephan. VitaCarn.

Mead Johnson
(Nutritional Division of Bristol Myers)
2404 Pennysylvania St.
Evansville, IN 47721

Enteral: Casec. Criticare HN. Isocal, Isocal HCN, Isocal II. Lonalac. MCT Oil. Moducal. Portagen. Sustacal, Sustacal HC. Susta II. Sustagen. Traumcal.

Feeding the Patient

Navaco Labs
  (Division of Lifetime
  Industries, Inc.)
4854 Research Dr.
San Antonio, TX 78240

Enteral: Intralife. Isolife. Pro-Mix. High Fat (MCT) Supplement. Pure Carbohydrate Supplement.

Norwich Eaton
  Pharmaceuticals Inc.
  (A Procter & Gamble Co.)
17 Eaton Ave.
Norwich, NY 13815

Enteral: Vivonex T.E.N., Tolerex.

Ross Laboratories
  (Div. of Abbott Labs.)
625 Cleveland Ave.
Columbus, OH 43216

Enteral: Enrich. Ensure, Ensure HN, Ensure Plus, Ensure Plus HN. Glucerna. Jevity. Osmolite, Osmolite HN. Polycose. ProMod. Pulmocare. Ross SLD. TwoCal HN. Vital HN.

Sandoz Nutrition
  (Clinical Products
  Division)
5320 W. 23rd St.
Minneapolis, MN 55416

Enteral: Citrotein. Compleat Regular, Compleat Modified. Isotein HN. Meritene. Nutrisource: Amino Acids, BCAA, Carbohydrate, Lipid LCT, Lipid MCT, Protein. Precision HN, Precision Isotonic, Precision LR. Resource, Resource Plus, Resource Instant Crystals. Stresstein.

Sherwood Medical
1831 Olive St.
St. Louis, MO 63103

Enteral: Attain, Attain LS, Pre-Attain. Comply. Magnacal. Microlipid. Pepti 2000. Propac. Sumacal. Vitaneed.

Note: Most of the above companies market their own feeding tubes and enteral/parenteral feeding devices, commonly referred to as **pumps** (see pages 70, 103).

LEGEND FOR ABBREVIATIONS

BCAA	= branched-chain amino acids	LS	= low sodium
HBC	= high branched-chain (amino acids)	MCT	= medium-chain triglycerides
HC	= high calorie	PC	= pure carbohydrate
HCN	= high calorie, high nitrogen	RF	= renal formulation
HN	= high nitrogen	SLD	= surgical liquid diet
LC	= liquid carbohydrate	STD	= standard diet
LCT	= long-chain triglycerides	T.E.N.	= total enteral nutrition
LR	= low residue		

CHAPTER 5
COMMENTS OF CLINICAL IMPORTANCE

NUTRITIONAL SCREENING

Usually the need for nutritional assessment in overnourished or undernourished patients is obvious. For example, there is the obese patient who frequently has placed himself or herself on peculiar, faddish reducing diets, resulting in protein malnutrition in the presence of excessive calories. On the other hand, there is the protein-calorie-deficient patient with chronic bowel disease, multiple trauma, sepsis, extensive surgery, or bone marrow transplantation ... and the list goes on. But there is a group of poorly nourished, *hospitalized patients* who somehow go unrecognized and untreated!

A quick look at the blood count and SMA 12/60, or simply taking a dietary history, may prove rewarding. *The following cardinal signals may alert the medical staff that nutritional assessment of the patient is indicated:* (1) poor appetite, (2) alcohol abuse, (3) progressive or recent weight loss, (4) weakness or apathy, (5) a serum albumin below 3.5 g/dl, or (6) a total lymphocyte count below 1800/microliter. Other readily available indicators seen in malnutrition are a serum cholesterol below 150 mg/dl (chronic liver disease must be ruled out) a BUN less than 10 mg/dl, and a serum phosphorus under 2.5 mg/dl (hypophosphatemia is also found in diabetes, hyperparathyroidism, alkalosis, and antacid therapy). *And finally, on physical examination, deficiencies in fat-soluble and water-soluble vitamins may produce the following signs:* (1) *HAIR*: alopecia, dryness, brittleness, easy pluckability; (2) *EYES*: night blindness, Bitot's spots, keratomalacia (softening of the cornea), angular palpebritis, xerophthalmia (dry eyeball); (3) *SKIN*: follicular hyperkeratosis, xerosis (dry skin), petechiae, ecchymosis, hyperpigmentation; (4) *MOUTH*: cheilosis (red, swollen, cracked lips), angular stomatitis, bleeding or receding gums, glossitis, magenta tongue, mucosal pallor; (5) *SKELETAL*:

osteomalacia, genu valgum (knock-knees), genu varum (bow-leg); and (6) *GENERAL*: edema, anemia, hepatomegaly, cardiomegaly, enlarged thyroid, loss of knee and ankle jerks.

Metabolic Responses to Critical Illness

(1) **Starvation (Figure 19).** Cahill's classic paper on starvation[168] emphasizes several salient points. First, when man is deprived of food, *the two main sources of fuel are triglyceride and muscle protein.* Second, man has three patterns of utilizing fuel:

  (a) **Combustion of glucose.** This oxidative reaction occurs chiefly in the brain and terminates with the production of CO_2 and H_2O. Thus, the fuel is spent and is no longer available as an energy source.

  (b) **Glycolysis.** The breakdown of sugar occurs primarily in the red blood cells but also in the white blood cells, bone marrow, renal medulla, and peripheral nerves. The end products, namely lactate and pyruvate (plus alanine), can then be remade in the liver into new glucose (gluconeogenesis) by energy from the oxidation of fat. The course of events involved in the rebirth of glucose as a source of fuel involves the recycle of carbon skeletons from glycolysis and is referred to as the **"Cori cycle."** The net effect is to spare protein.

  (c) **Utilization of fatty acids and ketones.** The two organic compounds fatty acids and ketone bodies serve as a source of fuel for the rest of the body including the heart, skeletal muscle, and kidney cortex. As fasting progresses, the brain adapts to using ketones (acetoacetate and b-hydroxybutyrate) as fuel, thus sparing protein. (Ketogenesis is inhibited during the stress-starvation state).

  (d) **Other major metabolic changes during starvation**
   i. O_2 uptake, REE, and insulin levels are lowered; glucagon levels are raised.
   ii. Fat is mobilized (lipolysis) with an increased output of free fatty acids (FFAs) and glycerol.
   iii. Muscle protein undergoes proteolysis to provide amino acid substrates (alanine, glutamine, leucine, isoleucine, valine) for gluconeogenesis (Alanine is the preferred amino acid substrate for hepatic gluconeogenesis).

Comments of Clinical Importance

BODY METABOLISM DURING FASTING

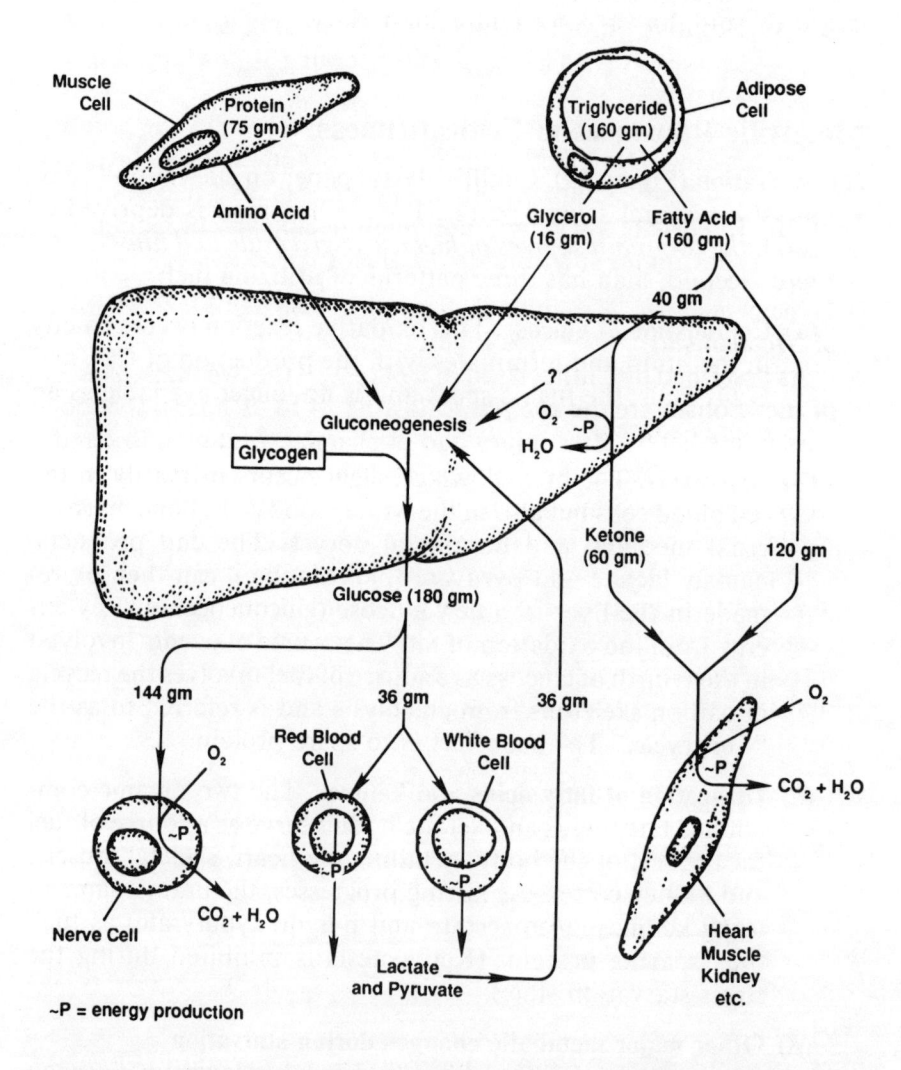

Figure 19. This drawing shows the biochemical adjustments made by a normal person who has been on an 1800 Calorie diet and starts to fast. From Jenkinson SG: Nutritional supplementation during mechanical ventilation. *In* Goldman AL (ed): *Problems in Pulmonary Disease* 3 (2): 1–8, Summer 1987; Newsletter by Bristol Laboratories, Copyright by PH Publishing Co, New York, NY 10003, with permission.

iv. Visceral protein becomes a fuel source as starvation progresses.
v. Negative nitrogen balance may eventually decline to as little as −3 to −4 g/day, thus conserving as much protein as possible.
vi. Natriuresis occurs during the first week following abrupt fasting. Decreases occur in levels of total body water, potassium, sodium, calcium, phosphorus, and magnesium.
vii. In *chronic* starvation, the renal metabolism of glutamine contributes substantially to glucose production.[169]

(2) Hypometabolism, Hypermetabolism (the "Ebb and Flow" Phases of Metabolism)[114,170-182] See Figures 3, 6.

As described by Cuthbertson in 1942,[171,172] the two main phases of metabolism are the *ebb phase* (lasting 24 to 48 hours) that occurs immediately after injury and is characterized by a lowered metabolic rate, and the subsequent *flow phase* (lasting days to weeks) that is accompanied by an elevated metabolic rate and depletion in body protein. *The flow phase has been* subdivided into four periods.[183] (1) a catabolic response to injury lasting 3–7 days (e.g., elective surgery) or longer (e.g., serious injury or sepsis), (2) a period of gradual improvement characterized by a reduction in nitrogen excretion and weight loss, (3) an anabolic response that may last for weeks, and (4) a final period during which there is restoration of fatty tissue.

(a) **Shock.** The disorder known as shock is the classic ebb phase of body metabolism.[173] Because of low cardiac output and resulting tissue hypoperfusion, O_2 uptake is lowered and fat metabolism (FFA turnover) is reduced.[173,182] *The main energy sources in shock are CHO and PRO rather than FAT.*

Cycle). Muscle protein is fragmented into amino acids which enter into the process of gluconeogenesis. In **prolonged** starvation (longer than 5–7 days) FAT becomes the predominant source of calories, thus sparing protein. The fat stores are mobilized as triglycerides, which are broken down into glycerol and free fatty acids. Glycerol is changed in the liver into glucose, and the fatty acids are partially oxidized to produce ketones. The heart, kidney cortex, and skeletal muscle use either fatty acids or ketone bodies for energy. As starvation continues, the brain adapts to utilizing ketones (in the absence of glucose) as fuel. In **late** starvation, as the fat stores are used up, muscle and visceral protein loss becomes critical. Death usually occurs from multiple organ failure after 50–60 days of starvation.

(b) **Trauma, Sepsis, Burns.**[114,173] A hypermetabolic state of the flow phase is seen in patients with mild to moderate trauma, early sepsis, or thermal injury, and can also follow stabilization of a patient who has been in shock. *The principal metabolic abnormalities are*
  (i) O_2 uptake and REE are increased.[173,174]
  (ii) Glucagon, glucocorticoids, catecholamines, glucose, vasopressin, growth hormone, ketone, and lactate levels are all elevated.[170-176]
  (iii) Gluconeogenesis is increased.[177,178]
  (iv) Insulin resistance develops.[173-179]
  (v) Nitrogen loss is increased, promptly resulting in a negative nitrogen balance. **Note:** Nitrogen loss is further accelerated if starvation (or semi-starvation) is imposed on a critical illness.[170,171,173]
  (vi) Amino acids are mobilized from skeletal muscle protein (proteolysis) with a rise in plasma concentrations of BCAA (leucine, isoleucine, valine).
  (vii) Lipolysis is increased, accompanied by a rise in serum levels of FFA and glycerol.[180] **Note:** Fat is the major source of energy in the hypermetabolic state. As much as 70%–90% of REE may come from the oxidation of fat with a decrease in RQ to 0.7–0.8.[152,173,181]

TYPES OF MALNUTRITION[184-188]

Although the following classification of malnutrition has been called too simplistic, it is useful to review the three types: (1) Calorie malnutrition (adult marasmus), (2) Protein malnutrition (adult kwashiorkor-like state), and (3) Calorie-protein malnutrition (marasmus-kwashiorkor mixture).

(1) Adult Marasmus (Cachexia).[18,184,186] The term "marasmus" literally means wasting away and applies to patients with chronic wasting of muscle mass and loss of subcutaneous fat due to insufficient intake of calories. The condition often is seen in patients following gastrectomy or in those with anorexia nervosa, dumping syndromes, obstructing gastric tumors, and carcinoma of the esophagus. *Whereas anthropometric measurements (Table 11) are abnormally decreased, measurements of visceral protein (Table 12) are preserved until the percent of ideal body weight falls below 85%.* Notwithstanding, depletion of visceral protein (with decreased resistance to infection and loss of immune response) occurs much more rapidly when stress is superimposed on an already semi-starved patient.

(2) Adult Kwashiorkor-like State.[18,185,186] The term kwashiorkor-like is applied to adult patients who have severe protein starvation without an appreciable decrease in their caloric intake. In fact, obesity may be present! Originally the disorder was described in young African Gold Coast children who, upon being taken off human milk, were fed foods high in carbohydrate and very low in protein content. The term stems from the native designation for "red boy" since the hair often changed to a streaky red hue.[188] *Kwashiorkor is characterized by a depletion of visceral protein stores, yet sufficient fat reserves and skeletal muscle mass are maintained.* Typically, laboratory tests reveal lowered values for serum albumin, TIBC, transferrin, and lymphocytes, plus decreased immune competence (Table 12). Anthropometric measurements are maintained. Overnourished adult patients with acute illness or significant injury are especially prone to develop a kwashiorkor-like state if given IV 5% dextrose for a long period of time. In children, kwashiorkor often is seen in those who are chronically ill secondary to disorders of maldigestion or malabsorption of the gut.

(3) Marasmus-Kwashiorkor Mixture.[186] This combined form of protein-calorie malnutrition often develops in critically ill, catabolic patients with trauma, sepsis, burns, or extensive surgery. As a group, these patients are prone to rapidly develop kwashiorkor-like hypoalbuminemia (serum albumin 2.5 g/dl or less), accompanied by edema of the GI tract and a protein-losing enteropathy.[189] Generally, the acute condition responds well to early intervention with a high nitrogen, peptide-based diet (low in fat) that is easily absorbed via the gut and results in rapid correction of the hypoalbuminemia without having to resort to IV albumin or TPN.[190] Otherwise, nutrition must be given by central vein to meet total energy requirements and to reverse a negative nitrogen balance.

POTPOURRI

ANTHROPOMETRY

(1) In the clinical setting, serial upper arm anthropometry (TSF, MAC, MAMC), as described on pages 17–20, will yield useful data. A thorough nutritional workup is indicated for persons with

values approaching the lower end of the scale at 5% (usually malnutrition) or the upper end of the scale at 95% (usually obesity). Other causes for extremes in these measurements (percentile distributions) are related to stature, edema, and state of health.

(2) Arm muscle circumference is the best available measurement of protein-calorie malnutrition (PCM). Unlike albumin, MAMC can mean only protein depletion since it is not primarily affected by kidney, liver, or GI disease.[191]

ENERGY, FUEL, STARVATION

(1) Energy can be neither created nor destroyed. The amount of energy (calories consumed) must be balanced with the calories that are burned, or body weight will change.[6]

(2) Resting energy expenditure (REE) represents the major portion of total energy expenditure in hospitalized patients.[2]

(3) For each 1° F elevation in body temperature, the resting energy expenditure will increase by approximately 7%.[10]

(4) During starvation, energy is first derived (for 1–2 days) from glycogen stored in the liver (22 g) and muscle (80 g) and next from the oxidation of free fatty acids (the major energy source during prolonged starvation). Then, after fat depletion, the major fuel source is protein in skeletal muscle and visceral organs.[192,193]

(5) In *chronic starvation,* the loss of body fat exceeds the loss of cell mass in a 2 to 1 ratio, but in *acute starvation* in a critically ill patient, this ratio may reverse to as low as 1 to 4 (Insel J, Elwyn DH: Body composition. *In:* Askanazi J, Starker P, Weissman C, eds. *Fluid and Electrolyte Management in Critical Care Patients.* Boston, Butterworths, 1986, pp. 3–38).

(6) Figure 19, page 114, shows that during starvation glucose is utilized by the brain, red and white blood cells, bone marrow, peripheral nerves, and renal medulla.[194] These obligate glucose-consuming tissues require 600–1000 kcal/day of glucose.[193] The glucose used by the brain is completely oxidized to CO_2 and H_2O. The other glycolytic tissues convert glucose primarily into lactate and pyruvate, which are then returned to the liver to be remade into glucose. The energy for this conversion is derived from the oxidation of fat. The net effect is to spare protein until the fat stores are gone.[194]

Comments of Clinical Importance

(7) In an adult of normal weight, the total energy available from food stores is around 1000–1200 kcal from CHO (only a small amount of glycogen is stored in the body), 130,000–160,000 kcal from fat (stored as triglyceride in adipose cells and broken down to glycerol and free fatty acids) and approximately 25,000–40,000 kcal from protein. The breakdown of lean body mass (muscle, viscera) results in loss of function.[5,192,193] Weakening of the diaphragm becomes a vital issue in patients on ventilators.

(8) Weight loss and serum albumin levels are two of the most important variables to evaluate the nutritional status of the patient.

(9) The dangers of overfeeding are just as real as underfeeding.

PROTEIN (PRO), NITROGEN BALANCE

(1) PRO is *functional* (muscle, organs, immune system) and is *not* intended to be used as a source of energy. On the other hand, CHO and FAT are natural, readily available sources of body fuel. Unfortunately, when energy intake is inadequate, the body draws not only on FAT but also PRO.

(2) In protein-calorie malnutrition (stress/starvation states), cannibalization of the diaphragm may contribute significantly to the onset of respiratory failure and also impede attempts to wean patients from mechanical ventilation.

(3) The human body can synthesize the nonessential but not the essential amino acids! Thus, the biosynthesis of a protein requires that all essential amino acids be included simultaneously in the diet, otherwise the patient will develop a negative nitrogen balance.[195] The essential amino acids for humans are valine, leucine, isoleucine, methionine, threonine, lysine, phenylalanine, and tryptophan. Histadine is essential for infants.

(4) Periodic determination of the patient's nitrogen balance will help to provide dynamic assessment of catabolism and PRO replacement.

(5) An increase in positive nitrogen balance without an increase in total energy intake (kcal/day) does not automatically equate with an improved nutritional response. For example, giving excessive amounts of amino acids (nitrogen) to thermally injured patients, will cause a protein-calorie mismatch which is manifested by increases in BUN levels out of proportion to serum creatinine con-

centrations. This complication is best handled by either reducing the intake of nitrogen or increasing the nonprotein calories (depending upon the total energy requirements of the individual).

LIPID EMULSIONS (FAT)

(1) Abnormalities in pulmonary gas exchange (DLco, PaO_2, $P[A-a]O_2$)* have been reported in patients receiving intravenous fat emulsions,[196-199] but in general have not been severe enough to be clinically significant. This phenomenon is most likely to occur in patients who already have damaged alveolar capillary membranes as in ARDS (adult respiratory distress syndrome). In fact, adequate oxygenation (to prevent O_2 desaturation) should be provided patients suffering from ARDS during fat emulsion therapy (Venus B, et al: Chest 95 (6): 1278-1281, 1989).

(2) The apparent lung dysfunction described above in item (1) is caused by changes in pulmonary vascular tone (from the fat-emulsion-related increase in prostaglandin production), resulting in mismatching of ventilation and perfusion. Skeie and colleagues[200] have pointed out that the increased synthesis of prostaglandins, which occurs from the polyunsaturated fatty acids in the intravenous fat emulsions, may have a therapeutic potential as modulators of immune and inflammatory responses.

(3) Prior to giving fat emulsions at our medical center, a baseline triglyceride value is obtained. Hyperlipidemia should clear before the next infusion. To avoid the "fat overload syndrome" one should closely monitor the plasma lipid profile, hemogram, blood coagulation, liver function tests, and platelet count (especially in the newborn).

(4) Rapid administration of lipid emulsion may cause fat and fluid overloading. The end result is overhydration due to increased endogenous production of water, dilution of serum electrolyte concentrations, dilutional anemia, pulmonary edema, impaired lung DLco (diffusing capacity), and metabolic acidosis.

(5) Great caution should be exercised in giving lipid emulsions to patients with severe liver or lung disease, anemia, coagulopathy, or a danger of fat embolism.

*DLco = diffusing capacity of the lung using carbon monoxide, single breath.
PaO_2 = partial pressure of oxygen in arterial blood.
$P(A-a)O_2$ = alveolar-arterial O_2 tension difference.

(6) Clinically, the manifestations of essential fatty acid deficiency (EFAD) are loss of hair, scaly dermatitis, retardation of growth, poor wound healing, fatty liver, and thrombocytopenia.

VITAMINS, MINERALS, WATER, OSMOLARITY

(1) *Vitamins and minerals* should be given to the patient in amounts sufficient to meet U.S. RDAs (Recommended Dietary Allowances)[119] as discussed on pages 98–100. Make certain that potassium, phosphorus, and magnesium needs are being met, especially in anabolic patients where these elements are incorporated into the synthesis of new body protein (e.g., 3 mEq of potassium are required per gram of nitrogen.[201])

(2) *The macrominerals are* potassium (k), sodium (Na), chloride (Cl), phosphorus (P), calcium (Ca), and magnesium (Mg).

(3) *The microminerals include* chromium (Cr), copper (Cu), manganese (Mn), selenium (Se), and zinc (Zn). These trace minerals are considered to be essential, along with iron, iodine, and cobalt. Other microminerals are fluorine (F), cadmium (Cd), molybdenum (Mo), vanadium (V), silicon (Si), and nickel (Ni).

(4) *Fluid requirements* must be monitored and fluids given or restricted as needed. Dehydration is common in the elderly, in persons on diuretics, and in the comatose patient who cannot express thirst. On the other hand, overhydration is common in the stressed patient. Also edema is frequently seen in the first two weeks of refeeding. Under ordinary circumstances, 1 ml of H_2O/Cal is adequate.[202] For normal persons, the daily water requirements can be calculated as being equal to 1500 ml H_2O/m^2 (where m^2 = square meters body surface area), or to an average value of 32 ml H_2O/kg.[203] Urinary output should be 1.5 to 2 times the renal solute load (the solutes are primarily Na, K, Cl, and urea). Note that insensible water loss increases greatly in patients with diarrhea, fever, and burns.

(5) *Osmolarity* is measured as mOsm/L and is defined as follows:[204]

$$\frac{\text{Concentration (mg/dl)} \times 10 \times N}{\text{atomic weight}}$$

where N = number of ionized particles per mole. For dextrose, N = 1, and the atomic weight of dextrose monohydrate is 198.17. Since 5% dextrose has 50 g/L (5000 mg/dl), the osmolarity is 252.3 mOsm/L.

Comments of Clinical Importance

(6) *Make certain* that the osmolality of a liquid diet is not too high.[55] Moderate osmolality (475–500 mOsm/kg H_2O) will minimize gastrointestinal distress. If osmolality is above moderate levels, then the liquid diet is diluted to at least one-half the original concentration to promote tolerance. Subsequently, the concentration can be increased as indicated.

RESPIRATORY QUOTIENT (RQ)

(1) Measuring the RQ (and energy expenditure) by indirect calorimetry may provide essential information to assist in weaning patients from mechanical ventilators and in managing COPD patients in a rehabilitation program.[77,78]

(2) Significant shifts in RQ are chiefly related to the energy substrates CHO and FAT. The various substrates being oxidized, caloric yields, and corresponding RQs are shown in Table 1, page 3.

(3) Excessive energy intake in any form (overfeeding) will promote **lipogenesis** and raise the RQ above 1.0.

(4) *As the RQ rises above 0.87, and especially over 1.0, there is an increasing ventilatory load that makes it difficult to wean ventilator-dependent patients.*

(5) In instances of overfeeding, downward adjustment of the total energy intake (kcals/day) may be all that is necessary to lower the RQ to acceptable levels.

(6) If the preceding maneuver (item 5) is not successful, then the CHO intake should be lowered and the proportion of FAT raised. *Notwithstanding, the FAT intake should not exceed 50%–60% of the total caloric value.*

(7) By following the ratio of CO_2 production to O_2 uptake, one can balance the CHO and FAT substrates to produce an ideal RQ in the range of 0.8 to 0.85.

(8) To achieve a desirable RQ in moderate to severe stress (hypermetabolic situations), a commonly used TPN regimen is to have 20%–25% of the total kcals/day as crystalline amino acids, then to render the remaining calories a 60/40 to 50/50 nonprotein mixture of dextrose and lipid emulsion. *In late sepsis or shock, however, FAT is **not** given except for enough essential fatty acids (EFAs) to prevent EFA deficiency.*

DRUG REACTIONS AND INTERACTIONS

Critically ill patients on multidrug therapy are at increased risk for drug-nutrient interactions. Schifferdecker and co-workers (*J Crit Illness* 4 [12]: 27–31, 1989) point out that micronutrients (K, Ca, P, HCO_3) may become chelated to form drug-nutrient complexes. The drug reactions and interactions listed below have been reviewed in detail by these authors (See Table 16, p. 124).

(1) The use of sodium polystyrene sulfonate (a cation-exchange resin) may induce hypokalemia, hypocalcemia, sodium retention, and fecal impaction. This product, when used in combination with aluminum hydroxide, may cause intestinal obstruction and metabolic alkalosis.

(2) Sodium citrate, in fresh frozen plasma and whole blood, can chelate calcium and also induce a metabolic alkalosis.

(3) Neomycin and many of the cephalosporins may interfere with the availability of vitamin K, leading to hypoprothrombinemia.

(4) The following drugs are capable of producing metabolic acidosis and hyperkalemia: aminoglycoside antibiotics, acetazolamide (diamox®), aldosterone antagonists, and IV hydrochloric acid. Amphotericin B also may cause a metabolic acidosis but potassium levels are lowered rather than raised. Note: Keep in mind that metabolic acidosis may be the result of a small bowel diarrhea due to the loss of bicarbonate.

(5) The following drugs are capable of producing metabolic alkalosis: furosemide, thiazides, carbenicillin, gluco- and mineralocorticoids, sodium bicarbonate, Ringer's lactate solution, acetate (hemodialysis, TPN), and citrate (blood products). Other precipitating factors may be loss of chloride by vomiting, nasogastric suctioning, and stool losses (e.g., large bowel diarrhea, short bowel syndrome). Also metabolic alkalosis may be seen in magnesium deficiency and severe hypokalemia ($K < 2$ mEq/L).

(6) The following drugs are capable of interfering with GI motility: atropine, morphine, hydroxyzine (atarax®, vistaril®), and diphenhydramine (benadryl®).

(7) Cisplatin and cyclosporine may induce large losses of magnesium in the urine due to renal tubular damage.

Table 16. SELECTED METHODS FOR CORRECTING DRUG-NUTRIENT PROBLEMS

Condition	Agent	Route	Dosage Range
Adicemia	Sodium acetate	I.V.	1-2 mEq/kg/d
	Sodium bicarbonate	Oral	1-2 mEq/kg/d (1 tsp = 60 mEq)
Alkalemia	Sodium chloride*	I.V.	Depends on serum levels
	Potassium chloride*	I.V.	Depends on serum levels
	Hydrochloric acid**	I.V.	1-2 mEq/kg/d
	Cimetidine	I.V.	900-1,200 mg/d
	Calcium chloride†	Oral	50 mEq/d
Hypocalcemia	Calcium chloride	I.V.	18-27 mEq/d
	Calcium gluconate	I.V.	18-27 mEq/d
	Calcium carbonate††	Oral	50-100 mEq/d
Hypokalemia	Potassium chloride	I.V.	Depends on serum levels
	Potassium phosphate	I.V.	Depends on serum levels
	Potassium chloride	Oral	Depends on serum levels
Hyponatremia	Sodium chloride	I.V.	Depends on serum levels
	Sodium chloride	Oral	Depends on serum levels (1 tsp = 85 mEq)
Hypophosphatemia	Sodium phosphate	I.V.	Up to 0.96 mmol/kg/d
	Potassium phosphate	I.V.	Up to 0.96 mmol/kg/d
	Neutra-Phos°	Oral	Up to 0.96 mmol/kg/d
Hypoprothrombinemia	Vitamin K	Subc.	Three 10-mg doses (acute); 5 mg 2 × wk for maintenance
	Vitamin K	Oral	5 mg/d (acute); 5 mg 2 × wk for maintenance.

*For mild hypochloremic metabolic alkaloses.
**For steroid-associated and severe metabolic alkalosis (pH > 7.50).
†Use only for acute hypocalcimia by separate bolus injection.
††The product Tums® contains 10 mEq/tablet.
°Contains 7 mmol of phosphorus/capsule.
NOTE: Cimetidine is used when large-volume nasogastric losses occur (significant losses of acid and chloride).

Adapted from Schifferdecker C, Driscoll DF, Bistrian BR: Management guidelines when drugs and nutrients interact, *J Crit Illness* 5 (1): 34–41, 1990, with permission.

(8) Corticosteroids may induce phosphaturia, as well as hypokalemia and metabolic alkalosis.

(9) Serum phosphorus (P) may be significantly reduced by the administration of nonabsorbable antacids (e.g., aluminum hydroxide). Also P levels may be lowered by insulin, hypertonic dextrose, and by conversion of the patient from a catabolic to anabolic state (P is transferred into the cells).

NUTRITIONAL ASSESSMENT

(1) For nutritional assessment, the results obtained by indirect calorimetry may be expressed as a percentage of Harris and Benedict's predicted REE, the normal range being 90%–100%. In this manner the individual can be classified as being hypometabolic, normometabolic, or hypermetabolic.[205]

(2) The nutritional needs of critically ill patients must be continuously monitored throughout the periods of stress and recovery since their energy expenditures may change rapidly, necessitating adjustments in calories and nitrogen.

(3) In critical care situations, TPN can correct (in most instances) protein-calorie malnutrition. A successful program involves closely following the patient, assessing and managing nutritional requirements, checking central lines for infection, monitoring volume status, electrolytes, glucose, lipid levels, liver function tests, acid-base balance, etc., and administering essential vitamins, minerals, and trace elements.

(4) *The bottom line in nutritional assessment: For accuracy, the energy requirements and substrate mixture in patients (especially those critically ill) must be measured since prediction equations are unreliable.*[16] *Not only does* **indirect calorimetry** *provide extremely useful information, but the procedure is cost-effective.*

TEAM APPROACH

A shocking fact is that malnutrition exists in our hospital patient population! Up to 50% of all hospitalized patients have been shown to suffer some degree of malnutrition, and 5% to 10% are severely malnourished.[18,35,206] Somehow, these people "slip through the cracks" and are not aggressively treated for their nutritional deficits. To solve the problem, a core group of interested professionals may organize a **hospital support team** whose purpose is to identify those patients with nutritional deficits (e.g., protein-calorie malnutrition) and to establish a nutritional program that offers safe, optimum nutritional support, in-house training, education, consultation services and quality control. Such programs using the team concept have proven to be self-supporting within 6 to 12 months. *For more detailed information, the reader is referred to a first-rate monograph titled "Establishing a Nutritional Support Service," 1980, Abbott Laboratories, North Chicago, Illinois, 60064. The ideal support team is comprised as follows:*

MEMBERS OF THE TEAM	RESPONSIBILITIES
1. Physician:	Serves as director of the service, is responsible for clinical aspects of nutritional support, provides consultation and in-house education and training.
2. Dietitian:	Performs nutritional assessments, follows the patient's status (energy requirements, nitrogen balance, etc.), assists physicians in nutritional management of their patients, formulates special enteral solutions, and carries out in-house teaching.
3. Nurse-Clinician:	Monitors the patient's clinical condition, coordinates nursing care for enteral and parenteral feedings, assists the physician in inserting intravenous feeding lines, and educates patients and their families regarding feedings at home.
4. Pharmacist:	Prepares feeding solutions (enteral and parenteral formulations) as required, provides in-service education, monitors the patient's progress, assures quality control, and assists in training patients for home feeding programs.
5. Surgeon:	Carries out catheter insertion for enteral feedings (PEG/PEJ tubes) and TPN. *Note:* The gastroenterologist also performs percutaneous endoscopic gastrostomy/jejunostomy.

6. Technician:	Performs indirect calorimetry on patients selected for nutritional studies. The services most often involved are surgical intensive care, medical intensive care, hematology-oncology, and burn units.
7. Physical Therapist:	Develops suitable exercises for the patients.
8. Social Worker:	Gives psychological support to the patients and deals with their financial concerns.
9. Secretary:	Keeps accurate records and assures proper charging.

Note: Many of the nutritional support teams in the United States are listed in *Nutritional Support Services*.[207] The list is updated periodically. Some foreign country teams also are included.

SUMMARY

Proper dietary support is an essential part of intensive care, a setting where protein-calorie malnutrition is common. Often, critically ill patients (those with trauma, burns, sepsis, or disease) cannot or do not eat well enough to meet their energy needs, necessitating feedings by enteral or parenteral routes. Depending upon the patient's condition, different feeding techniques are utilized: (1) Insertion of a nasoenteric tube into the stomach or jejunum, (2) insertion of a PEG or PEJ tube via percutaneous endoscopic gastrostomy, and (3) cannulation of a peripheral or central vein.

For the past 70 years the Harris-Benedict prediction equation has been used to *estimate* the energy requirements of malnourished patients, often resulting in underfeeding or overfeeding in the critically ill patient. Today, indirect calorimetry can be used to accurately *measure* the patient's oxygen uptake ($\dot{V}O_2$), carbon dioxide production ($\dot{V}CO_2$), and the respiratory quotient ($RQ = \dot{V}CO_2/\dot{V}O_2$) in critical care situations. **The calculation for the resting energy expenditure is made by using Weir's conventional equation:**

REE = [3.914 ($\dot{V}O_2$) + 1.106 ($\dot{V}CO_2$) 1.44 − (2.17 UN),

where UN = total urinary nitrogen in grams/day, and REE = resting energy expenditure measured in kcals/day.

Using Weir's short equation:

REE = [3.9 ($\dot{V}O_2$) + 1.1 ($\dot{V}CO_2$)] 1.44.

Thus, by employing a metabolic cart one not only can determine the total energy needs of the individual but also adjust the energy substrates (CHO and FAT) to achieve an ideal RQ in the range of 0.8 to 0.87.

Regarding diet, sufficient glucose should be given to obtain a maximal protein-sparing effect and to supply the requirements of glucose dependent tissues. However, large amounts of CHO or excessive calories in any form (overfeeding) will promote lipogenesis, raise the RQ above 1.0, precipitate acute respiratory failure in severe COPD patients, and impair weaning in ventilator-dependent patients. Downward adjustment of the total amount of nutriment given to compromised lung patients with high RQs may be all that is necessary to lower the RQ to acceptable levels. If this maneuver is not successful, the CHO intake should be lowered and the proportion of FAT raised but not exceed 50%–60% of the total calories.

Nutritional support must also provide adequate amounts of PRO (the substrate for anabolism). The protein status of the patient can be evaluated by looking at the nitrogen balance, serum albumin, transferrin, total iron binding capacity, creatinine-height index, arm muscle circumference, total lymphocyte count, and skin tests for anergy. The triceps skinfold and lean body weight are useful measurements for appraising fat stores.

Conclusion

To successfully carry out nutritional assessment and feeding (enteral/parenteral) in critical care, the best approach is to utilize the skills of a *nutritional support team* consisting of the physician, surgeon, nurse-clinician, dietitian, pharmacist, and technician. The combination of anthropometry, appropriate biochemical tests, and indirect calorimetry ($\dot{V}O_2$, $\dot{V}CO_2$, RQ) enables one to precisely assess the metabolic status of the patient, the total energy requirement (kcals/day), and the correct substrate mixture. The essential key, previously lacking, is gas exchange monitoring by indirect calorimetry, which has proven to be accurate and cost-effective! *Of the many prediction equations to estimate the resting energy expenditure, none are as reliable as indirect calorimetry in determining the energy needs of most patients.*

REFERENCES

(1) French SN: Nutritional assessment via indirect calorimetry. Tech Notes, Medical Graphics Corporation, St. Paul, MN, 1987.

(2) Elwyn DH, Kinney JM, Askanazi J: Energy expenditure in surgical patients. Surg Clin North Am 61 (3): 545–556, 1981.

(3) Boothby WM, Sandiford I: *Laboratory Manual of the Technique of Basal Metabolic Rate Determinations,* Philadelphia, WB Saunders Co., 1920, pp. 11, 24.

(4) Benedict FG, Carpenter TM: Metabolism and energy transformation of healthy man during rest. Washington DC, Carnegie Institute, 1910, publication no. 126.

(5) Krause MV, Mahan LK: *Food, Nutrition and Diet Therapy,* 7th edition. Philadelphia, WB Saunders Co., 1984, pp. 9–23.

(6) Long CL, Blakemore WS: Energy and protein requirements in the hospitalized patient. JPEN 3 (2): 69–71, 1979.

(7) Long CL, Schaffel N, Geiger JW, et al: Metabolic response to injury and illness: Estimation of energy and protein needs from indirect calorimetry and nitrogen balance. JPEN 3 (6): 452–456, 1979.

(8) Wolfe RR: Carbohydrate metabolism in the critically ill patient. Crit Care Clinics 3 (1): 11–24, 1987.

(9) Kinney JM: Energy metabolism. *In* Fisher JE (ed), *Surgical Nutrition.* Boston; Little, Brown & Co., 1983, p. 99.

(10) DuBois EF: *Basal Metabolism in Health and Disease,* 2nd edition. Philadelphia, Lea & Febiger, 1927, pp. 112–127.

(11) Blackburn GL, Maini BS, Bistrian BR, et al: Surgical nutrition, *In* Halpern SL (ed), *Clinical Nutrition,* 2nd edition, Philadelphia, JB Lippincott Co, 1987, pp. 170–194.

(12) Krause MV, Mahan LK: *Food, Nutrition, and Diet Therapy,* 7th edition. Philadelphia, WB Saunders Co., 1984, p. 12.

(13) Kinney JM: *In* Ballinger WF, Collins JA, Drucker WR (eds): *Manual of Surgical Nutrition,* Philadelphia, WB Saunders Co., 1975, 223–235.

References

(14) Anderson CE: Energy and Metabolism, *In* Schneider HA, Anderson CE, Coursin DB (eds): *Nutritional Support of Medical Practice,* Hagerstown, MD, Harper & Row Publishers, 1977, p. 12.

(15) Zavala DC: *Manual on Exercise Testing: A Training Handbook,* 2nd edition. Iowa City, Department of Publications, The University of Iowa, 1987, pp. 93-98.

(16) Foster GD, Knox LS, Dempsey DT, et al: Caloric requirements in total parenteral nutrition. J Am College Nutr 6 (3): 231-253, 1987.

(17) Clouse RE: Parenteral nutrition. *In* Wyngaarden JB, Smith LH Jr (eds), *Cecil Textbook of Medicine,* 18th edition. Philadelphia, WB Saunders Co., 1988, pp. 1247-1251.

(18) Blackburn GL, Bistrian BR, Maini BS, et al: Nutritional and metabolic assessment of the hospitalized patient. JPEN 1: 11-22, 1977.

(19) Bernard MA, Jacobs DO, Rombeau JL: *Nutritional and Metabolic Support of Hospitalized Patients.* Philadelphia, WB Saunders Co., 1986.

(20) Frisancho AR, Flegal PN: Relative merits of old and new indices of body mass with reference to skinfold thickness. Am J Clin Nutr 36 (4): 697-699, 1982.

(21) Zavala DC, Printen KJ: Basal and exercise tests on morbidly obese patients before and after gastric bypass. Surgery 95 (2): 221-229, 1984.

(22) National Center for Health Statistics. Plan and operation of the Health and Nutrition Examination Survey, United States, 1971-1973. Rockville, MD: National Center for Health Statistics, 1979. Vital and health statistics. Series 1: Programs and collection procedure, No. 10a. DHEW Publ. No. (PHS) 79-1310.

(23) Bishop CW, Bowen PE, Ritchey SJ: Norms for nutritional assessment of American adults by upper arm anthropometry. Am J Clin Nutr 34: 2530-2539, 1981.

(24) Bishop CW, Ritchey SJ: Evaluating upper arm anthropometric measurements. J Am Dietetic Assn 84 (3): 330-335, 1984.

(25) Gray GE, Gray LK: Validity of anthropometric norms used in the assessment of hospitalized patients. J Parent Ent Nutr 3 (5): 366-368, 1979.

(26) Weight by Height and Age for Adults 18-74 Years: United States, 1971-1974. Vital and Health Statistics. Series 11: Data from the National Health Survey, No. 208. DHEW Publ. No. (PHS) 79-1656.

(27) Kaminski MV Jr, Jeejeebhoy KN: Nutritional assessment-Diagnosis of malnutrition and selection of therapy. *In* Tuckerman MM, Turco SJ (eds), *Human Nutrition.* Philadelphia, Lea & Febiger, 1983, pp. 189-214.

(28) Forbes G, Bruining GJ: Urinary creatinine excretion and lean body mass. Am J Clin Nutr 29: 1359–1366, 1976.

(29) Sauberlich HE, Skala JH, Dowdy RP: *Laboratory Tests for the Assessment of Nutritional Status.* Cleveland, OH, CRC Press Inc, 1974.

(30) Assessment of Protein Nutritional Status: A Committee Report. Am J Clin Nutr 23: 807–819, 1970.

(31) Bistrian BR, Blackburn GL, Sherman M, et al: Therapeutic index of nutritional depletion in hospitalized patients. Surg Gyn Obstet 141: 512–516, 1975.

(32) Harper HA: *Review of Physiological Chemistry,* 16th edition, Los Altos, Lang Medical Publications, 1975.

(33) Garb S: *Laboratory Tests in Common Use,* 6th edition, Springer Publishing Co, 1970.

(34) Bistrian BR, Blackburn GL, Hallowell E, et al: Protein status of general surgical patients. JAMA 230: 858–860, 1974.

(35) Bistrian BR, Blackburn GL, Vitale J, et al: Prevalence of malnutrition in general medical patients. JAMA 235: 1567–1570, 1976.

(36) Kernstine, KH, Cerra FB, Buchwald H: Enteral and parenteral nutrition. *In* Halpern SL (ed), *Quick Reference to Clinical Nutrition,* 2nd edition. Philadelphia, JB Lippincott Co, 1987, pp. 324–355.

(37) Bistrian BR, Blackburn GL, Scrimshaw NS, et al: Cellular immunity in semi-starved states in hospitalized adults. Am J Clin Nutr 28: 1148–1155, 1975.

(38) Tayek JA, Blackburn GL: Goals of nutritional support in acute infections. Am J Med 76: 81–90, 1984.

(39) Lutwak L: Evaluation of Nutritional status. *In* Halpern SL (ed), *Quick Reference to Clinical Nutrition,* 2nd edition. Philadelphia, JB Lippincott Co, 1987, pp. 1–11.

(40) Schade AL, Caroline L: An iron-binding component in human blood plasma. Science 104: 340–341, 1946.

(41) Katz JH: Iron and protein kinetics studied by means of doubly labelled human crystalline transferrin. J Clin Invest 40: 2143–2152, 1961.

(42) Tamburro CH: Nutritional management of alcoholism, drug addiction, and acute toxicity syndromes. *In* Halpern SL (ed), *Quick Reference to Clinical Nutrition,* 2nd edition. Philadelphia, JB Lippincott Co, 1987, pp. 430–456.

(43) Stromberg BV, Davis RJ, Danziger LH: Relationship of serum transferrin to total iron binding capacity for nutritional assessment. JPEN 6 (5): 392–394, 1982.

References

(44) Miller SF, Morath MA, Finley RK: Comparison of derived and actual transferrin: A potential source of error in clinical nutritional assessment. J Trauma 21 (7): 548–550, 1981.

(45) Ingenbleek Y, De Visscher M, De Nayer P: Measurement of prealbumin as an index of protein-calorie malnutrition. Lancet 2: 106–109, 1972.

(46) Ingenbleek Y, Van Den Schrieck HG, De Nayer P, et al: The role of retinol-binding protein in protein calorie malnutrition. Metabol 24 (5): 633–641, 1975.

(47) Smith FR, Suskind R, Thanangkul O, et al: Plasma vitamin A, retinol-binding protein and prealbumin concentrations in protein-calorie malnutrition. Response to varying dietary treatments. Am J Clin Nutr 28 (7): 732–738, 1975.

(48) Igenbleek Y, Van Den Schrieck HG, De Nayer P, et al: Albumin, transferrin and the thyroxine-binding prealbumin/retinol-binding protein (TBPA-RBP) complex in assessment of malnutrition. Clin Chem Acta 63 (1): 61–67, 1975.

(49) Blackburn GL, Williams LF, Bistrian BR, et al: New approaches to the management of severe acute pancreatitis. Am J Surg 131:114–124, 1976.

(50) Law DK, Dudrick SJ, Abdou NI: Immunocompetence of patients with protein-calorie malnutrition. The effects of nutritional repletion. Ann Intern Med 79: 545–550, 1973.

(51) Nielsen HJ, Hammer JH, Moesgaard F, et al: Ranitidine prevents postoperative transfusion-induced depression of delayed hypersensitivity. Surg 105 (6): 711–717, 1989.

(52) Mac Burney M, Wilmore DW: Rational decision-making in nutritional care. Surg Clin N Amer 61: 571–582, 1981.

(53) Kaminski MV Jr: Enteral hyperalimentation. Surg Gyn Obstet 143: 12–16, 1976.

(54) Kaminski MV Jr: Parenteral hyperalimentation technique. Am J IV Therapy, December–January, 1975.

(55) Maillet JO: Calculating parenteral feedings: A programmed instruction. Amer Dietetic Assn 84 (11): 1312–1323, 1984.

(56) Lindeman RD: Minerals in medical practice. *In* Halpern SL (ed), *Quick Reference to Clinical Nutrition,* 2nd edition. Philadelphia, JB Lippincott Co, 1987, pp. 295–323.

(57) Massry SG: The clinical syndrome of phosphate depletion. Adv Exp Med Biol 103: 301–312, 1978.

(58) Jaun D, Elrazak MA: Hypophosphatemia in hospitalized patients. JAMA 242: 163–164, 1979.

(59) Deitel M, Williams VP, Rice TW: Nutrition and the patient requiring mechanical ventilatory support. J Am Coll Nutr 2: 25–32, 1983.

(60) Newman JH, Neff TA, Ziporin P: Acute respiratory failure associated with hypophosphatemia. N Eng J Med 296: 1101–1103, 1977.

(61) Klock JC, Williams HE, Mentzer WC: Hemolytic anemia and somatic cell dysfunction in severe hypophosphatemia. Arch Intern Med 134: 360–364, 1974.

(62) Juan D: The causes and consequences of hypophosphatemia. Surg Gynecol Obstet 153: 589–597, 1982.

(63) Lau K: Phosphate disorders. *In* Kokko JP, Tannen RL (eds): *Fluids and Electrolytes,* 1st edition, Philadelphia, WB Saunders, 1986, pp. 398–471.

(64) Baker JP, Lemoyne M: Nutritional support in the critically ill patient: If, when, how, and what. Crit Care Clinics 3 (1): 97–113, 1987.

(65) Zaloga GP: Interpretation of the serum magnesium level. Chest 95 (2): 257–258, 1989.

(66) Caddell JL: The magnesium load test, I: A design for infants. Clinical Pediatrics 14: 449–451, 457–459, 518–519, 1975.

(67) Quebbeman EJ, Ausman RK: Estimating energy requirements in patients receiving parenteral nutrition. Arch Surg 117: 1281–1284, 1982.

(68) Harris JA, Benedict FG: A Biometric Study of Basal Metabolism in Man. Washington DC, Carnegie Institute, 1919 (publication No. 279).

(69) Feurer ID, Mullen JL: Measurement of energy expenditure. *In* Rombeau J, Caldwell M (eds), *Clinical Nutrition (Vol. 2): Parenteral Nutrition.* Philadelphia, WB Saunders Co., 1986, pp. 224–236.

(70) Chumlea WC, Roche AF, Mukherjee D: *Nutritional Assessment of the Elderly Through Anthropometry,* Columbus, OH, Ross Laboratories, 1987, p. 40.

(71) Cerra F: *Pocket Manual of Surgical Nutrition.* St. Louis, CV Mosby Co, 1984.

(72) Moore JA, Angelillo VA: Prediction equation to determine REE (Resting Energy Expenditure) in ambulatory patients with moderate to severe COPD. Chest 92 (supplement): S1295, 1987 (abstract).

(73) Curreri PW, Richmond D, Marvin J, et al: Dietary requirements of patients with major burns. J Am Diet Assn 65: 415–417, 1974.

(74) Pearson E, Soroff HS: Burns. *In* Schneider HA, Anderson CE, Coursin DB (eds), *Nutritional Support of Medical Practice.* Hagerstown, MD, Harper & Row Publishers, 1977, pp. 222–235.

(75) Lund CC, Browder NC: The estimation of areas of burns. Surg Gynecol Obstet 79: 352–358, 1944.

References

(76) Pruitt BA Jr, Goodwin CW Jr: Burns: Including cold, chemical and electrical injuries. *In* Sabiston DC Jr (ed), *Textbook of Surgery,* 13th edition, Vol. 1. Philadelphia, WB Saunders Co., 1986, pp. 215–216.

(77) Mann S, Westenskow DR, Houtchens BA: Measured and predicted caloric expenditure in the acutely ill. Crit Care Med 13 (3): 173–177, 1985.

(78) Carlsson M, Nordenstrom J, Hedenstierna G: Clinical implications of continuous measurement of energy expenditure in mechanically ventilated patients. Clin Nutr 3: 103–110, 1984.

(79) Gassaniga AB, Polachek JR, Wilson AF, et al: Indirect calorimetry as a guide to caloric replacement during total parenteral nutrition. Am J Surg 136: 128–133, 1978.

(80) Saffle JR, Medina E, Raymond J, et al: Use of indirect calorimetry in the nutritional management of burned patients. J Trauma 25: 32–39, 1985.

(81) Turner WW, Ireton CS, Hunt JL: Predicting energy expenditure in burned patients. J Trauma 25: 11–16, 1985.

(82) Clifton GL, Robertson CS, Choi SC: Assessment of nutritional requirements of head-injured patients. J Neurosurg 64: 895–901, 1986.

(83) Weir JB de V: New methods for calculating metabolic rate with special reference to protein metabolism. J Physiol (London) 109: 1–9, 1949.

(84) Wilmore DW: *The Metabolic Management of the Critically Ill.* New York, Plenum Publishing Corp, 1977, p. 16.

(85) Swinamer DL, Phang PT, Jones RL, et al: Twenty-four hour energy expenditure in critically ill patients. Crit Care Med 15 (7): 637–643, 1987.

(86) Hannenberg S, Soderberg D, Groth T, et al: Carbon dioxide production during mechanical ventilation. Crit Care Med 15: 3–13, 1987.

(87) Eccles RC, Swinamer DL, Jones RL, King G: Validation of a compact system for measuring gas exchange. Crit Care Med 14 (9): 802–811, 1981.

(88) Weissman C, Kemper M, Damask MC, et al: Effect of routine intensive care interactions on metabolic rate. Chest 86 (6): 815–818, 1984.

(89) Askanazi J, Nordenstrom J, Rosenbaum SH, et al: Nutrition for the patient with respiratory failure. Anesthesiology 54 (5): 373–377, 1981.

(90) Elwyn DH, Gump FE, Munro HN, et al: Changes in nitrogen balance of depleted patients with increasing infusions of glucose. Am J Clin Nutr 32: 1597–1611, 1979.

(91) Kinney JM, Morgan AP, Domingues FJ, et al: A method for continuous measurement of gas exchange and expired radioactivity in acutely ill patients. Metabolism 13: 205–211, 1964.

(92) Spencer JL, Zikria BA, Kinney JM, et al: A system for continuous measurement of gas exchange and respiratory functions. J Appl Physiol 33: 523–528, 1972.

(93) Feurer I, Currier G, Mullen J: Reliability of indirect calorimetric measurements via two gas collection techniques: canopy and mouthpiece. Proceedings of the 7th Congress of the European Society of Parenteral and Enteral Nutrition, 159, 1985.

(94) Browning J: The effects of fluctuating FIO_2 on metabolic measurements in the mechanically ventilated patient. Crit Care Med 10: 82–85, 1982.

(95) Dietrich KA, Romero MD, Conrad SA: The technique of measuring energy expenditure at the bedside. J Crit Illness 4 (7): 65–74, 1989.

(96) Bishop MJ, Benson MS, Pierson DJ: Carbon dioxide excretion via bronchopleural fistulas in adult respiratory distress syndrome. Chest 91 (3): 400–402, 1987.

(97) Lewis WD, Chwals W, Benotti PN, et al: Bedside assessment of the work of breathing. Crit Care Med 16 (2): 117–122, 1988.

(98) Brinson RR: Enteral nutrition in the critically ill patient: The role of hypoalbuminemia. *In* Roche AF (ed): *The Gastrointestinal Response to Injury, Starvation, and Enteral Nutrition,* Report of the Eighth Ross Conference on Medical Research. Columbus, Ohio, Ross Laboratories, 1988, pp. 59–61.

(99) Selivanon V, Sheldon G: Enteral nutrition and sepsis. *In* Rombeau J, Caldwell M (eds): *Enteral and Tube Feeding.* Philadelphia, WB Saunders, 1984, pp. 403–411.

(100) Orr G, Wade J, Bothe A, et al: Alternatives to total parenteral nutrition in the critically ill patient. Crit Care Med 8: 29–34, 1980.

(101) Rolandelli RH, Koruda MJ, Guenter P, Rombeau JL: Enteral nutrition: Advantages, limitations, and formula selection. J Crit Illness 3 (10): 93–106, October, 1988.

(102) Rolandelli RH, Koruda MJ, Guenter P, Rombeau JL: Techniques for administering enteral nutrition in the ICU. J Crit Illness 3 (10): 107–112, October, 1988.

(103) Rombeau JL, Caldwell MD (eds), *Clinical Nutrition: Enteral and Tube Feeding.* Philadelphia, WB Saunders, 1984.

(104) Silk DBA, Rees RG, Keohane PP, et al: Clinical efficacy and design changes of "fine bore" nasogastric feeding tubes: A seven year experience involving 809 intubations in 403 patients. JPEN 11: 378–383, 1987.

(105) Cataldi-Beltcher EL, Seltzer MH, Slocum BA, et al: Complications occurring during enteral nutritional support: A prospective study. JPEN 7: 546–552, 1983.

(106) Roubenoff R, Ravich WJ: The technique of avoiding feeding tube misplacement. J Crit Illness 4 (8): 75–79, 1989.

(107) Berger R, Adams L: Nutritional support in the critical care setting (Part 2). Chest 96 (2): 372–380, 1989.

(108) Wasiljew BK, Ujiki GT, Beal JM: Feeding gastrostomy: Complications and mortality. Am J Surg 143 (2): 194–195, 1982.

(109) Ruge J, Vasquez RM: An analysis of the advantages of Stamm and percutaneous endoscopic gastrostomy. Surg Gynecol Obstet 162: 13–16, 1986.

(110) Gauderer MWL, Ponsky JL, Izant RJ: Gastrostomy without laparotomy: A percutaneous endoscopic technique. J Pediatr Surg 15: 872–875, 1980.

(111) Larson DE, Burton DD, Schroeder KW, et al: Percutaneous endoscopic gastrostomy: Indications, success, complications, and mortality in 314 consecutive patients. Gastroenterol 93: 48–52, 1987.

(112) Jain NK, Larson DE, Schroeder KW, et al: Antibiotic prophylaxis for percutaneous endoscopic gastrostomy. Ann Intern Med 107: 824–828, 1987.

(113) Pingleton SK, Hodzima SK: Enteral alimentation and gastrointestinal bleeding in mechanically ventilated patients. Crit Care Med 11: 13–16, 1983.

(114) Koruda MJ, Guenter P, Rombeau JL: Enteral nutrition in the critically ill. Crit Care Clinics 3 (1): 133–153, 1987.

(115) Garg A, Bonanome A, Grundy SM, et al: Comparison of a high-carbohydrate diet with a high-monounsaturated-fat diet in patients with non-insulin-dependent diabetes mellitus. N Engl J Med 319 (13): 829–834, 1988.

(116) Davidson MB, Peters AL, Isaac RM: Lack of glucose rise after simulated tube feeding with a low carbohydrate, high fat enteral formula in Type I diabetic patients. Clinical Research 37: 140A, 1989.

(117) Silberman H, Dixon NP, Eisenberg D: The safety and efficacy of a lipid-based system of parenteral nutrition in acute pancreatitis. Am J Gastroenterol 77: 494–497, 1983.

(118) Stegink LD: Amino acids in pediatric parenteral nutrition. Am J Dis Child 137: 1008–1016, 1983.

(119) Annan GL: An exhibition of books on the growth of our knowledge of blood transfusion. Bull NY Acad Med 15: 622–632, 1939.

(120) Latta T: Saline venous injection in cases of malignant cholera performed while in the vapour-bath. Lancet 1: 173–174, 208–209, 1832–1833.

(121) Biedl A, Kraus R: Uber intravenose Traubenzucherinfusionen an Menschen. Wien Klin Wochenschr 9: 55–65, 1986.

(122) Abderhalden E, Rona P: Futterungsversuche mit durch Pankreatin durch Pepsinsalzaire plus Pankreatin und durch Saure hydrolysiertem Casein. Hoppe Seylers Z Physiol Chem 42: 528–539, 1904.

(123) Henriques V, Andersen AC: Uber parenterale Ernahrung durch intravenose Injektion. Hoppe Seylers Z Physiol Chem 88: 357–369, 1913.

(124) Holt LR Jr, Tidwell HC, McNair Scott TFS: The intravenous administration of fat: A practical therapeutic procedure. J Pediatr 6: 151–160, 1935.

(125) Elman R: Intravenous injection of amino acids in regeneration of serum protein following severe experimental hemorrhage. Proc Soc Exp Biol Med 36: 867–870, 1937.

(126) Elman R, Weiner DO: Intravenous alimentation with special reference to protein (amino acid) metabolism. JAMA 112: 796–802, 1939.

(127) Shohl AT, Butler AM, Blackfan KD, et al: Nitrogen metabolism during oral and parenteral administration of the amino acids of hydrolyzed casein. J Pediatr 15: 469–475, 1939.

(128) Kinney JM: Nutrition in the intensive care patient. Crit Care Clinics 3 (1): 1–10, 1987.

(129) Schoenheimer R, Rittenberg D; Study of intermediary metabolism of animals with aid of isotopes. Physiol Rev 20: 218–248, 1940.

(130) Helfrick FW, Abelson NM: Intravenous feeding of a complete diet in a child: Report of a case. J Pediatr 25: 400–403, 1944.

(131) Mueller JF: Symposium on intravenous fat emulsions. Am J Clin Nutr 16: 1–3, 1965.

(132) Olson GB, Teasley KM, Cerra FB: Balanced parenteral nutrition. Nutritional Support Services 5 (6): 16–20, 1985.

(133) Jeejeebhoy KN: *Role of Fat in Parenteral Nutrition.* Chicago, Medical Directions, Inc, 1980.

(134) Dudrick SJ, Rhoads JE, Vars HM, et al: Growth of puppies receiving all nutritional requirements by vein. Fortschr Parenteral Ernahr 2: 16–18, 1967.

(135) Wilmore DW, Dudrick SJ: Growth and development of an infant receiving all nutrients exclusively by vein. JAMA 203: 860–864, 1968.

References

(136) Dudrick SJ, Wilmore DW, Vars HM, et al: Can intravenous feeding as a sole means of nutrition support growth in the child and restore weight loss in an adult? An affirmative answer. Ann Surg 169: 974–984, 1969.

(137) Wilmore DW, Groff DB, Bishop HC, et al: Total parenteral nutrition in infants with catastrophic gastrointestinal anomalies. J Pediatr Surg 4: 181–189, 1969.

(138) Dudrick, SJ: The genesis of intravenous hyperalimentation. JPEN 1 (1): 23–29, 1977.

(139) Meng HC: Parenteral nutrition: Principles, nutrient requirements, techniques, and clinical applications. In Schneider HA, Anderson CE, Coursin DB (eds), *Nutritional Support of Medical Practice*. Hagerstown, MD, Harper & Row Publishers, 1977, pp. 152–183.

(140) Daly JM, Masser E, Hansen L, et al: Peripheral vein infusion of dextrose/amino acid solutions, +/− 20% fat emulsion. JPEN 9 (3): 296–299, 1985.

(141) Orme JF Jr., Clemmer TP: Meeting nutritional needs during mechanical ventilation. J Respir Dis 12: 35–40, 1985.

(142) Jensen GL, Bistrian BR: Total parenteral nutrition: Which formulation for which patients? J Crit Illness 4 (2): 78–86, 1989.

(143) McCarthy MC, Shives JK, Robinson RJ, et al: Prospective evaluation of single and triple lumen catheters in total parenteral nutrition. JPEN 11 (3): 259–262, 1987.

(144) Jensen GL, Bistrian BR: Techniques for administering total parenteral nutrition. J Crit illness 4 (2): 87–93, 1989.

(145) Bone RC: The techniques of subclavian and femoral vein cannulation. J Crit Illness 3 (7): 61–68, July 1988.

(146) Vander Salm TJ: Internal jugular vein cannulation. In Vander Salm TJ (ed), *Atlas of Bedside Procedures*. Boston, Little, Brown & Co Inc, 1979, pp. 37–46.

(147) Freis ES: Vascular cannulation. In Kofke WA, Levy JH (eds), *Postoperative Critical Care Procedures of the Massachusetts General Hospital*. Boston, Little, Brown & Co Inc, 1986, pp. 125–139.

(148) Scott WL: Complications associated with central venous catheters: A survey. Chest 94 (6): 1221–1224, 1988.

(149) Jensen GL, Bistrian BR: Techniques for preventing and managing complications of TPN. J Crit Illness 4 (3): 79–87, 1989.

(150) Bivins BA, Hyde GL, Sachatello CR, et al: Physiopathology and management of hyperosmolar hyperglycemic nonketotic dehydration. Surg Gynecol Obstet 154 (4): 534–540, 1982.

(151) Wolfe RR, O'Donnell TF Jr, Stone MD, et al: Investigation of factors determining the optimal glucose infusion rate in total parenteral nutrition. Metabolism 29 (9): 892–900, 1980.

(152) Askanazi J, Carpentier YA, Elwyn DH, et al: Influence of total parenteral nutrition on fuel utilization in injury and sepsis. Ann Surg 191: 40–46, 1980.

(153) Askanazi J, Elwyn DH, Silverberg PA, et al: Respiratory distress secondary to a high carbohydrate load: A case report. Surgery 87: 596–598, 1980.

(154) Askanazi J, Rosenbaum SH, Hyman AI, et al: Respiratory changes induced by the large glucose loads of total parenteral nutrition. JAMA 243: 1444–1447, 1980.

(155) Fisher JE: Nutritional support in the seriously ill patient. Curr Probl Surg 17: 466–532, 1980.

(156) Askanazi J, Weissman C, LaSala PA, et al: Effect of protein intake on ventilatory drive. Anesthesiology 60: 106–110, 1984.

(157) Abbott WC, Grakauskas AM, Bistrian BR, et al: Metabolic and respiratory effects of continuous and discontinuous lipid infusions. Arch Surg 119: 1367–1371, 1984.

(158) Adamkin DH, Gelke KN, Andrews BF: Fat emulsions and hypertriglyceridemia. JPEN 8 (5): 563–567, 1984.

(159) Hallberg D: Studies on the elimination of exogenous lipids from the blood stream. The kinetics for the elimination of chylomicrons studied by single intravenous injections in man. Acta Physiol Scand 65: 279–284, 1965.

(160) Brown RO, Heizer WD: Nutrition and respiratory disease. Clin Pharm 3 (2): 152–161, 1984.

(161) Mok KT, Maiz A, Yamazaki K, et al: Structured medium-chain and long-chain triglyceride emulsions are superior to physical mixtures in sparing body protein in the burned rat. Metabolism 33 (10): 910–915, 1984.

(162) National Research Council, Food and Nutrition Board: *Recommended Dietary Allowances,* 9th ed. Washington DC, National Academy of Sciences, 1980, pp. 33–35.

(163) Jeejeebhoy KN, Chu RC, Marliss EB, et al: Chromium deficiency, glucose intolerance and neuropathy reversed by chromium supplementation, in a patient receiving long-term total parenteral nutrition. Am J Clin Nutr 30 (4): 531–538, 1977.

(164) Abumrad NN, Schneider AJ, Steel D, et al: Amino acid intolerance during prolonged total parenteral nutrition reversed by molybdate therapy. Am J Clin Nutr 34 (11): 2551–2559, 1981.

References

(165) Driscoll DF, Baptista RJ, Bistrian BR, et al: Practical considerations regarding the use of total nutrient admixtures. Am J Hosp Pharm 43 (2): 416–419, 1986.

(166) Al-Jurf AS, Younoszai H: *Total Parenteral Nutrition: Policies, Procedures, and Prescribing Information.* Iowa City, IA, University of Iowa Hospitals and Clinics publication (monograph), 1989.

(167) Bern MM, Bothe A Jr, Bistrian B, et al: Prophylaxis against central vein thrombosis with low-dose warfarin. Surgery 99 (2): 216–221, 1986.

(168) Cahill GF: Starvation in man. N Engl J Med 282: 668–675, 1970.

(169) Cahill GE, Aoki TT: Renal gluconeogenesis and amino acid metabolism in man. Med Clin North Am 59 (3): 751–761, 1975.

(170) Baker JP, Lemoyne M: Nutritional support in the critically ill patient: If, when, how, and what. Crit Care Clin 3 (1): 97–113, 1987.

(171) Cuthbertson DP: Post shock metabolic response. Lancet 1: 433–437, 1942.

(172) Cuthbertson DP: The metabolic response to injury and its nutritional implications: Retrospect and prospect. JPEN 3: 108–129, 1979.

(173) Wiener M, Rothkopf MM, Rothkopf P, et al: Fat metabolism in injury and stress. Crit Care Clinics 3 (1): 25–56, 1987.

(174) Long CL, Schaffel N, Geiger JW, et al: Metabolic response to injury and illness: Estimation of energy and protein needs from indirect calorimetry and nitrogen balance. JPEN 3: 452–456, 1979.

(175) Davies CL, Newman RJ, Molyneux SG, et al: The relationship between plasma catecholamines and severity of injury in man. J Trauma 24: 99–105, 1984.

(176) Gerich JE, Lorenzi J, Bier DM, et al: Effects of physiologic levels of glucagon and growth hormone on human carbohydrate and lipid metabolism. J Clin Invest 57: 875–884, 1976.

(177) Long CL, Kinney JM, Geiger JW: Nonsuppressibility of gluconeogenesis by glucose in septic patients. Metabolism 25: 193–201, 1976.

(178) Elwyn DH, Kinney JM, Jeevanandam M, et al: Influence of increasing carbohydrate intake on glucose kinetics in injured patients. Ann Surg 190: 117–127, 1979.

(179) Black PR, Brooks DC, Bessey PQ, et al: Mechanism of insulin resistance following injury. Ann Surg 196: 420–435, 1982.

(180) Stoner HB, Frayn KN, Barton RN, et al: The relationships between plasma substrate and hormones and the severity of injury in 277 recently injured patients. Clin Sci 56: 563–573, 1979.

(181) Elwyn DH, Gump FE, Iles M, et al: Protein and energy sparing of glucose added in hypocaloric amounts to peripheral infusions of amino acids. Metabolism 27: 325–331, 1978.

(182) Daniel AM, Pierce CH, Shizgal HM, et al: Protein and fat utilization in shock. Surgery 84: 588–594, 1978.

(183) Moore FD: *Metabolic Care of the Surgical Patient,* Philadelphia, WB Saunders, 1959.

(184) Bistrian BR, Blackburn GL, Vitale J, et al: Prevalence of malnutrition in general medical patients. JAMA 235: 1567–1570, 1976.

(185) Bistrian BR, Blackburn GL, Hallowell E, et al: Protein status of general surgical patients. JAMA 230: 858–860, 1974.

(186) Kaminski MV, Jeejeebhoy KN: Nutritional Assessment-Diagnosis of malnutrition and selection of therapy. *In* Tuckerman MM, Turco SJ (eds), *Human Nutrition.* Philadelphia, Lea & Febiger, 1983, pp. 189–214.

(187) Bistrian BR, Sherman M, Blackburn GL, et al: Cellular immunity in adult marasmus. Arch Intern Med 137 (10): 1408–1411, 1977.

(188) Scrimshaw NS, Behar M, Arroyave G, et al: Kwashiorkor in children and its response to protein therapy. JAMA 164: 555–561, 1957.

(189) Brinson RR: Enteral nutrition in the critically ill patient: The role of hypoalbuminemia. *In* Roche AF (ed): *The Gastrointestinal Response to Injury, Starvation, and Enteral Nutrition,* Report of the Eighth Ross Conference on Medical Research. Columbus, Ohio, Ross Laboratories, 1988, pp. 59–61.

(190) Brinson RR, Kolts BE: Diarrhea associated with severe hypoalbuminemia: A comparison of a peptide-based chemically defined diet and standard enteral alimentation. Crit Care Med 16 (2): 130–136, 1988.

(191) Blackburn GL, Bistrian BR: Nutritional support resources in hospital practice. *In* Schneider HA, Anderson CE, Coursin DB (eds): *Nutritional Support of Medical Practice,* Hagerstown, MD, Harper & Row Publishers, 1977, p. 147.

(192) Robin AP, Greig PD: Basic principles of intravenous nutritional support. Clinics in Chest Med 7 (1): 29–39, 1986.

(193) Kinney JM, Weissman C: Forms of malnutrition in stressed and unstressed patients. Clinics in Chest Med 7 (1): 19–28, 1986.

(194) Jenkinson SG: Nutritional supplementation during mechanical ventilation. Goldman AL (ed): Problems in Pulmonary Disease 3 (2): 1–8, summer, 1987.

References

(195) Thorp FK, Peirce P, Deedwania C: Nutrition in the infant and young child. *In* Halpern SL (ed), *Quick Reference to Clinical Nutrition,* 2nd edition, Philadelphia, JB Lippincott Co, 1987, p. 73.

(196) Greene HL, Hazlett D, Demaree R: Relationship between intralipid-induced hyperlipemia and pulmonary function. Am J Clin Nutr 29 (2): 127-135, 1976.

(197) Sundstrom G, Zauner CW, Arborelius M Jr: Decrease in pulmonary diffusing capacity during lipid infusion in healthy men. J Appl Physiol 34: 816-820, 1973.

(198) Talbott GD, Frayser R: Hyperlipidaemia: A cause of decreased oxygen saturation. Nature 200: 684, 1963.

(199) Venus B, Patel CG, Mathru M, et al: Pulmonary effects of lipid infusion in patients with acute respiratory failure. Crit Care Med 12 (3): 293, 1984 (abstract).

(200) Skeie B, Askanazi J, Rothkopf MM, et al: Intravenous fat emulsions and lung function: A review. Crit Care Med 16 (2): 183-194, 1988.

(201) Cannon PR, Frazier LE, Hughes RH: Influence of potassium on tissue protein synthesis. Metabolism 1: 49-57, 1952.

(202) Food and Nutrition Board, National Research Council: *Recommended Dietary Allowances,* 9th edition, Washington; National Academy of Sciences, 1980.

(203) Talbot NB, Kerrigan GA, Crawford JD, et al: Application of homeostatic principles to the practice of parenteral fluid therapy. N Engl J Med 252: 856-862, 898-906, 1955.

(204) MacBurney MM, Young LS: Formulas. *In* Rombeau JL, Caldwell MD (eds): *Clinical Nutrition: Enteral and Tube Feeding.* Philadelphia, WB Saunders, 1984, pp. 171-198.

(205) Feurer I, Mullen JL: Bedside measurement of resting energy expenditures and respiratory quotient via indirect calorimetry. Nutrition in Clin Practice 1: 43-49, 1986.

(206) Blackburn GL, Bistrian BR, Maini BS, et al: *Manual for Nutritional/Metabolic Assessment of the Hospitalized Patient.* Presented at the 62nd Annual Clinical Congress of the American College of Surgeons, Chicago, Oct. 11-15, 1976 (also see reference 16).

(207) Nutritional Support Services 7 (11): 29-59, 1987 (7628 Densmore Ave., Van Nuys, Ca 91406-9976).

INDEX

Abbott Laboratories, 108
Acidosis/Alkalosis. See *Metabolic acidosis/alkalosis.*
  See *Drug-nutrient problems.*
Acknowledgments (book), xiii–xiv
Activity factor, 37, 38, 42
Adenosine triphosphate (ATP), 3, 4
Albumin, 25, 26 (Table 12), 27
Alcoholism, 75, 77
Alpha Therapeutic Corp., 108
Alveolar-arterial oxygen difference [$P(A-a)O_2$], 120
Amino acids, 75, 76, 80, 94, 103, 104, 108, 109, 119
Amphotericin B, 123
Anabolism, 5
Anergy. See *Skin tests.*
Antacids,
  harmful interactions, 123
Antibiotics,
  harmful interactions, 123
Aspiration,
  prevention of, 71, 72

Basal energy expenditure (BEE), 9
Basal metabolic rate (BMR), 1, 2 (Fig. 1), 10
Biosearch Medical Products, Inc., 109
Blood urea nitrogen (BUN), 32, 34
Body frame type, 14 (Table 3)

Index

Body mass index (BMI). See *Body weight.*

Body mass, lean (LBM). See *Body weight.*

Body metabolism, 3, 4, 113, 115

Body surface area (BSA),
  measurement of, 6
  to predict resting energy expenditure (REE), 36

Body weight,
  body mass index (BMI), 13, 15
  ideal weight for height, 15, 16 (Table 4)
  ideal weight by rule of thumb, 16 (Table 5)
  lean body mass (LBM), 7
  percent of ideal weight (% IBW), 12
  percent of usual weight (% UBW), 13

Boehringer isolation valve, 57

Book order information, xv

Breath-by-breath analysis, 46, 56

Broviac catheter, 87

Bubble. See *Canopy.*

Burns,
  Curreri formula, 39
  energy requirements, 41
  feeding formulas, 76
  metabolic abnormalities, 116
  protein requirements, 41
  rule of nines, 40
  stress factor, 40

Cachexia. See *Marasmus.*

Calcium, 90, 91, 124 (Table 16)

Calculating parenteral feedings, 103–107

Caloric density, 91, 92 (Table 15)

Calorie malnutrition, 25 (Table 11)

Calorie/Nitrogen ratio (Cal/N), 8

Calorimetry,
  accessory devices, 51–55
  definition, 7
  direct calorimetry, 7
  equation, short, 43
  equation, Weir's, 42
  indirect calorimetry, 41–58
  manufacturers, 49, 50
  measurement conditions, 43–46
  mechanically ventilated patients, 56, 57

Index

operation, 47, 48
sources of error, 58, 59
quality control, 47, 48

Cannulation of central vein, 85, 86

Canopy, 46, 47 (Fig. 8a), 48 (Fig. 8b), 51, 55, 56 (Fig. 15)

Carbohydrate (CHO), 93, 126

Carbon dioxide production ($\dot{V}CO_2$), 7, 42–44, 126

Cardiac cachexia,
feeding formula, 78, 79
therapeutic modes, 78, 79

Carnitine, 95

Case study, 59–66

Catabolism, 5

Catheter (to cannulate central vein), 87 (Fig. 18),
Broviac, 87
complications of insertion, 86
Groshong, 87
Hickman, 87
multichannel type, 85
sepsis, 86

Cation-exchange resin, 123

Central venous nutrition (CVN). See *Total parenteral nutrition (TPN)*.
definition, 10

Chemical balance, 89

Cholesterol, 34

Classification of diets,
complete vs incomplete, 79, 80
composition, 74–79

Clintec Nutrition Co., 109

Computerized compounder, 101

Conclusion (book), 128

Contents (book), iii

Cori cycle, 113

Corticosteroids, 123

Creatinine-Height index (CHI), 20, 21, 23 (Table 9), 24 (Table 10)

Curreri equation, 39, 40

Diabetes,
special formula, 77

Diarrhea, 70

Drug-nutrient problems, 123, 124 (Table 16)

Diets,
   classification of, 74–80
   complete diets, 79, 80
   feedings used in case study, 62, 64
   incomplete diets, 80
   special formulas, 75–80

Dietary thermogenesis, 7

Diffusing capacity of lung (DLco), 120

Direct calorimetry. See *Calorimetry*.

Drug reactions/interactions, 123, 124 (Table 16)

Ebb phase. See *Hypometabolism*.

Electrolytes, 32, 33, 89–91, 97, 98

Energy,
   energy balance, 4 (Fig. 2)
   general information, 118
   energy needs, 9
   energy requirements (calculated REE), 35–40
   energy requirements (measured REE), 41–43

Enteral feeding/formulas, 74–80, 109, 110
   for cardiac cachexia, 78, 79
   for diabetes, 77
   for hepatic encephalopathy, 75
   for pancreatitis, 77, 78
   for renal failure, 75, 76
   for respiratory failure, 76, 77
   for stress/trauma/burns, 76
   modular, 75
   oligomeric, 74
   polymeric, 74
   special diets, 75–79

Enteral nutrition, 68–80

Equations. See *Prediction equations for REE*.
         See *Shortcut equations*.
         See *Weir's equations for REE*.

Essential fatty acids, (EFAs), 97, 121

Essential thermogenesis, 7

Essential trace metals. See *Trace metals*.

Extended TPN, 87 (Fig. 18), 88, 102, 103

External jugular vein. See *Jugular vein*.

Index

Fat (FAT). See *Lipid emulsions.*
  essential fatty acids (EFAs), 96, 121
  fatty acids/ketones, 113, 114 (Fig. 19)
  general information, 94–97
  hyperlipidemia, 95, 120
  infusion rates, 95
  linoleic acid, 96
  measurement of fat stores, 13 (Table 2)
  medium-chain triglycerides (MCTs), 96, 97
  overload syndrome, 120

Feeding pumps. See *Pumps.*

Feeding tube, 68. See *Nasoenteric tube feeding.*

Flow phase. See *Hypermetabolism.*

Fluid balance, 88, 121

Foreword (book), ix

Formulas. See *Diets.*
       See *Enteral formulas.*
       See *Parenteral formulas.*

Fuel,
  general comments, 118
  physiologic value for substrates, 1, 3 (Table 1)

Gambro Engstrom, 51, 54 (Fig. 13)

Gas sample line, 57 (Fig. 16)

Gastrostomy, 72, 73

Gastrointestinal tract,
  diarrhea, 70
  nausea and vomiting, 70
  steps to correct complications, 71, 72

Gluconeogenesis, 5

Glucose,
  combustion of, 113
  glycolysis, 113

Groshong catheter, 87

Hans Rudolph, Inc., 51, 55 (Fig. 14)

Harris-Benedict equation, 37, 38, 126

Heparin, 99

Hepatic encephalopathy,
  special feeding formula, 75

Hickman catheter, 87

Home TPN, 87 (Fig. 18), 102, 103
Hood. See *Canopy*.
Hyperglycemia, 70, 88, 93
Hypermetabolism, 115
Hypernatremia, 89, 90
Hypoalbuminemia,
 major causes of, 27
Hypocalcemia. See *Calcium*.
Hypokalemia. See *Potassium*.
Hypometabolism, 115
Hyponatremia, 90, 124 (Table 16).
Hypophasphatemia. See *Phosphorus*.
Hypoprothrombinemia, 124 (Table 16)

Indirect calorimetry. See *Calorimetry*.
Infusion rates/amounts, 92–96
Insulin, 93, 99
Internal jugular vein. See *Jugular vein*.
Introduction (book),
 to Chapter 1 (background information), 1–3
 to Chapter 4 (feeding the patient), 67, 68

Jugular vein (external/internal), 85, 86, 87 (Fig. 18)

KabiVitrum, Inc., 109
Kendall Mc Gaw Labs., Inc., 109
Ketones, 113, 114 (Fig. 19)
Kilocalorie, 8
Krause-Mahan equation, 36
Kwashiorkor, 117

Laboratory tests, 24, 25, 26 (Table 12), 27–33, 61–65 (case study)
Laminar flow hood, 101
Legend for enteral formula abbreviations, 111
Linoleic acid, 96, 97
Lipid emulsions,
 history of, 81, 82

Index

general comments, 94-97, 120, 121
marketing companies, 97, 108, 109

Lipoprotein lipase, 96

Long's calculations, 35

Lymphocyte count. See *Total lymphocyte count (TLC)*.

Magnesium (Mg), 33, 34, 121

Malnutrition. See *Calorie malnutrition*.
        See *Kwashiorkor*.
        See *Marasmus*.
        See *Marasmus-kwashiorkor*.
        See *Protein malnutrition*.

Manufacturers of metabolic carts, 49-50

Marasmus, 116

Marasmus-kwashiorkor, 117

Marketing companies for nutritional products, 108-111

Mask (mouth/face), 51, 55 (Fig. 14)

Mead Johnson, 109

Mechanical problems (feeding tube), 70

Medical Graphics Corp., 46 (Fig. 7), 47 (Fig. 8a), 48 (Fig. 8b), 49, 50 (Fig. 10), 51

Medium-chain triglycerides (MCTs), 96, 97

MET, 8

Metabolic acidosis/alkalosis, 89, 91, 123, 124 (Table 16)

Metabolic carts,
  accessory devices, 51-57
  equipment, 46 (Fig. 7), 47, 48, 50 (Fig. 10), 52 (Fig. 11), 53 (Fig. 12), 54 (Fig. 13)
  manufacturers, 49-50
  measurement conditions, 43-45
  operation/quality control, 47

Metabolic complications,
  due to drugs, 123
  during tube feedings, 70, 72
  during TPN, 88
  therapy of, 124 (Table 16)

Metabolism,
  breath-by-breath measurement on CRT screen, 49 (Fig. 9)
  definition, 3, 4
  responses to fasting/starvation, 113, 115

Metoclopramide, 74
Midarm circumference (MAC), 17–19, 20 (Fig. 5), 21 (Table 7)
Midarm muscle circumference (MAMC), 17–20, 22 (Table 8)
Modular formula, 75
Moore-Angelillo equation, 38, 39
Multitest (skin testing), 29
Multivitamins. See *vitamins*.

Nasoenteric tube feeding,
  complications, 70, 71
  contraindications, 69
  indications, 68, 69
  preventive measures, 71, 72
  techniques, 69, 70
Nausea/vomiting, 70
Navaco Labs, 110
Nitrogen,
  balance, 26 (Table 12), 29–32, 119, 120
  excretion, 30 (Fig. 6)
Norwich Eaton Pharmaceuticals, Inc., 110
Nurse-clinician, duties, 126
Nutrition,
  enteral, 68–80
  parenteral, 80–107
Nutritional assessment,
  case study, 59–66
  general comments, 11, 112, 125
  screening, 112
  support team, 125, 126, 127
Nutritional products, 108–110

Oligomeric formula, 74
Oral feeding, 67, 68
Osmolarity, 8, 83, 91, 121
Outline (book), v–viii
Oxygen uptake ($\dot{V}O_2$), 7, 42–44, 66, 126

Pancreatitis,
  special diet, 77, 78

Index

Parenteral formulas, 108, 109
  additives, 97–101
  calculations, 103–107
  carbohydrate (CHO), 93, 94
  concentrations, 91, 92
  electrolytes, 97, 98
  fat (FAT), 94–97
  heparin/insulin, 99
  infusion rates, 92, 93
  medium-chain triglycerides (MCTs), 96, 97
  minerals/trace metals, 99–101
  nutrient requirements, 93–97
  program at Iowa, 101–103
  protein (PRO), 94
  steps in preparing formulas, 103–107
  vitamins, 98, 99

Parenteral nutrition, 80–107. See *Total Parenteral Nutrition*.

Percutaneous endoscopic gastrostomy (PEG),
  complications, 72, 73
  general comments, 72, 73

Percutaneous endoscopic jejunostomy (PEJ), 73

Peripheral venous nutrition (PVN), 10, 82, 83

Pharmacist, duties, 101, 126

Phosphorus (P), 32, 33, 121, 123, 124 (Table 16)

Pneumotachometer, 58 (Fig. 17)

Pneumothorax, 86

Polymeric formula, 74

Potassium, 90, 124 (Table 16)

Potpourri, 117–124

Pre-albumin (PA), 28

Prediction equations for REE (resting energy expenditure),
  Body surface area, 36
  Curreri formula, 39, 40
  Harris-Benedict, 37, 38, 44 (Table 14)
  Krause-Mahan, 36
  Long's calculations, 35
  Moore-Angelillo, 38, 39
  Quebbeman-Ausman, 36

Prediction equations for transferrin, 26 (Table 12), 27

Preface (book), x

Protein (PRO),
  general information, 94, 119

Index

kwashiorkor, 117
malnutrition, 26 (Table 12), 117
nitrogen balance, 29–32
requirements (in burns), 41
skeletal protein status, 17–24, 25 (Table 11), 116
visceral protein status, 24, 25, 26 (Table 12), 27–29

Pumps (to deliver nutrients), 70, 103, 110

Quebbeman-Ausman equation, 36

Reading suggested, xii, 34, 107, 108
References (book), 130–143
Renal damage,
  by drug therapy, 123
Renal failure,
  equation adjustment for nitrogen balance, 32
  special diet/formulas, 75, 76
Respiratory quotient (RQ), 1, 3 (Table 1), 7, 122, 126
Resting energy expenditure (REE), 1, 2 (Fig. 1), 5 (Fig. 3), 10, 35–43, 44 (Table 14), 63, 127, 128
Retinol-binding protein (RBP), 28
Ross Laboratories, 110
RQ. See *Respiratory quotient.*
RQnp (non-protein RQ), 7
Rule of nines (burns), 40

Sandoz Nutrition, 110
SensorMedics Corp., 51, 52 (Fig. 11), 56 (Fig. 15)
Sepsis, 116
Sherwood Medical, 110
Serum albumin. See *Albumin.*
Shivering thermogenesis, 7
Shock, 115
Shortcut equations (for REE), 43, 44 (Table 14)
Skeletal muscle measurements, 13 (Table 2), 17, 18, 20–24
Skeletal protein status, 17–24, 25 (Table 11), 116
Skin tests (for anergy), 26 (Table 12), 29
Sodium/chloride, 89

Sodium polystyrene sulfate (resin), 123
Sodium restriction, 79
Solution mixtures (for TPN), 101, 102
Special Nitrogen balance equation (uremic patient), 32
Special formulas for feeding. See *Diets.*
                               See *Enteral formulas.*
                               See *Parenteral formulas.*

Specific dynamic action (Rubner). See *Dietary thermogenesis.*
Starvation, 113, 114 (Fig. 19), 118, 119
Stress factor, 37, 38, 39 (Table 13), 40
Stress levels, 84, 104
Stress/trauma/burns,
  hypermetabolic state, 116
  special feeding formula, 76
Subclavian vein, 85, 86, 87 (Fig. 18)
Substrate
  definition, 5
  fuel value, 1, 3 (Table 1)
Summary (book), 127, 128
Superior vena cava. See *Vena cava.*
Support team. See *Nutritional assessment.*
Surgeon, duties, 126

Team approach. See *Nutritional assessment, support team.*
Technician, duties, 127
Thermal injury. See *Burns.*
Thermogenesis,
  dietary, 1, 6
  essential, 6
  percent of TEE, 2 (Fig. 1)
  shivering, 6
Three-in-one system, 101
Total energy expenditure (TEE), 1, 2 (Fig. 1), 10
Total iron binding capacity (TIBC), 26 (Table 12), 27
Total lymphocyte count (TLC), 26 (Table 12), 28, 29
Total parenteral nutrition (TPN)
  additives, 97–101
  catheter care, 86

Index

    central venous route, 83–88
    complications, 86, 88–91
    extended TPN, 87, 88
    formulas/infusions, 91–103
    historical background, 80–82
    home TPN, 102–103
    indications, 83–85
    infusion devices (pumps), 103
    solution mixtures, 101, 102
    steps in calculating formulas, 103–107
    techniques in cannulation, 85, 86

Trace metals, 99–101

Transferrin, 26 (Table 12), 27, 28

Trauma, 116

Triceps skinfold (TSF), 17, 18 (Table 6), 19 (Fig. 4)

Tube feeding. See *Nasoenteric tube feeding.*

Uremia. See *Renal failure.*

$\dot{V}CO_2$. See *Carbon dioxide production.*

$\dot{V}O_2$. See *Oxygen uptake.*

Vein injury, 83, 86, 91

Vena cava, 85, 86, 87 (Fig. 18)

Visceral protein status, 24–32, 26 (Table 12), 117

Vitamins,
    content of Berocca, M.V.I.-12, 98, 99
    deficiencies (physical findings), 112, 113
    vitamin K, 99, 124 (Tabel 16)

Waters Instruments, Inc., 51, 53 (Fig. 12)

Weir's equations, 42, 43, 44 (Table 14), 127

White blood count, 28

FIGURES 1-19

Figure 1: Expenditure of Energy in Healthy Individuals, p. 2
Figure 2: Energy Balance, p. 4
Figure 3: Resting Energy Expenditure, p. 5
Figure 4: Triceps Skinfold Measurement, p. 19
Figure 5: Midarm Circumference Measurement, p. 20
Figure 6: Starvation vs Injury (Nitrogen Dynamics), p. 30
Figure 7: Metabolic Cart at the Bedside, p. 46
Figure 8: Medical Graphics Corporation Bubble/Hood, pp. 47, 48
Figure 9: Metabolic Study on CRT Screen, p. 49
Figure 10: Medical Graphics Corporation Critical Care Monitor, p. 50
Figure 11: SensorMedics Metabolic Monitor, p. 52
Figure 12: Waters Instruments Metabolic Monitoring System, p. 53
Figure 13: Gambro Engstrom Metabolic Unit, p. 54
Figure 14: Hans Rudolph "VOCA" Mouth/Face Mask, p. 55
Figure 15: SensorMedics Canopy-Blower System (Hood), p. 56
Figure 16: Gas Sample Line (Patient on Ventilator), p. 57
Figure 17: Pneumotachometer, p. 58
Figure 18: Central Venous Line for TPN, p. 87
Figure 19: Body Metabolism During Fasting, p. 114

TABLES 1-16

Table 1: Fuel Value and RQ of Major Nutrients, p. 3
Table 2: Nutritional Assessment, p. 13
Table 3: Body Frame Type, p. 14
Table 4: Ideal Weight for Height: Adults, pp. 15, 16
Table 5: Rule of Thumb Determination for Ideal Body Weight, p. 16
Table 6: Triceps Skinfold Data (Males/Females), p. 18
Table 7: Midarm Circumference Data (Males/Females), p. 21
Table 8: Midarm Muscle Circumference Data (Males/Females), p. 22
Table 9: 24-Hour Urinary Creatinine Excretion for Men, p. 23
Table 10: 24-Hour Urinary Creatinine Excretion for Women, p. 24
Table 11: Degree of Calorie Malnutrition, p. 25
Table 12: Degree of Protein Malnutrition, p. 26
Table 13: Levels of Stress and Nutritional Needs, p. 39
Table 14: Equations for Resting Energy Expenditure, p. 44
Table 15: Caloric Density of Venous Nutrient Substrates, p. 92
Table 16: Methods for Correcting Drug-Nutrient Problems, p. 124

Typesetting by:
Compositors Corporation
830 First Ave. N.E.
Cedar Rapids, Iowa 52402

NOTES